Evaluation and Management of Vulvar Disease

Editor

ARUNA VENKATESAN

OBSTETRICS AND GYNECOLOGY CLINICS OF NORTH AMERICA

www.obgyn.theclinics.com

Consulting Editor
WILLIAM F. RAYBURN

September 2017 • Volume 44 • Number 3

ELSEVIER

1600 John F. Kennedy Boulevard • Suite 1800 • Philadelphia, Pennsylvania, 19103-2899

http://www.theclinics.com

OBSTETRICS AND GYNECOLOGY CLINICS OF NORTH AMERICA Volume 44, Number 3
September 2017 ISSN 0889-8545, ISBN-13: 978-0-323-54562-4

Editor: Kerry Holland
Developmental Editor: Kristen Helm

Obstetrics and Gynecology Clinics (ISSN 0889-8545) is published quarterly by Elsevier Inc., 360 Park Avenue South, New York, NY 10010-1710. Months of issue are March, June, September, and December. Periodicals postage paid at New York, NY, and additional mailing offices. Subscription price per year is $301.00 (US individuals), $627.00 (US institutions), $100.00 (US students), $377.00 (Canadian individuals), $792.00 (Canadian institutions), $225.00 (Canadian students), $459.00 (international individuals), $792.00 (international institutions), and $225.00 (international students). To receive student/resident rate, orders must be accompanied by name of affiliated institution, date of term, and the signature of program/residency coordinator on institution letterhead. Orders will be billed at individual rate until proof of status is received. Foreign air speed delivery is included in all *Clinics* subscription prices. All prices are subject to change without notice. POSTMASTER: Send address changes to *Obstetrics and Gynecology Clinics*, Elsevier Health Sciences Division, Subscription Customer Service, 3251 Riverport Lane, Maryland Heights, MO 63043. **Customer Service: Telephone: 1-800-654-2452 (U.S. and Canada); 314-447-8871 (outside U.S. and Canada). Fax: 314-447-8029. E-mail: journalscustomerservice-usa@elsevier.com (for print support); journalsonlinesupport-usa@elsevier. com (for online support).**

Reprints. For copies of 100 or more of articles in this publication, please contact the Commercial Reprints Department, Elsevier Inc., 360 Park Avenue South, New York, New York 10010-1710. Tel.: 212-633-3874; Fax: 212-633-3820; E-mail: reprints@elsevier.com.

Obstetrics and Gynecology Clinics of North America is also published in Spanish by McGraw-Hill Interamericana Editores S.A., P.O. Box 5-237, 06500, Mexico; in Portuguese by Reichmann and Affonso Editores, Rio de Janeiro, Brazil; and in Greek by Paschalidis Medical Publications, Athens, Greece.

Obstetrics and Gynecology Clinics of North America is covered in MEDLINE/PubMed (Index Medicus), Excerpta Medica, Current Concepts/Clinical Medicine, Science Citation Index, BIOSIS, CINAHL, and ISI/BIOMED.

Contributors

CONSULTING EDITOR

WILLIAM F. RAYBURN, MD, MBA
Distinguished Professor, Emeritus Chair, Department of Obstetrics and Gynecology,
Associate Dean, Continuing Medical Education and Professional Development, University
of New Mexico School of Medicine, Albuquerque, New Mexico, USA

EDITOR

ARUNA VENKATESAN, MD, FAAD
Associate Chief of Service, Division of Dermatology, Santa Clara Valley Medical Center,
Clinical Associate Professor, Affiliated Department of Dermatology, Stanford University,
Stanford, California, USA

AUTHORS

JILL I. ALLBRITTON, MD
Dermatopathologist, Bethesda Dermpath Laboratory, Silver Spring, Maryland, USA;
Dermatologist, Anne Arundel Dermatology, Towson, Maryland, USA; Lecturer, Pathology,
Johns Hopkins University, Baltimore, Maryland, USA

TANJA G. BOHL, MBBS, FACD
Dermatologist, Vulva Clinic, Jean Hailes Medical Centre, Clayton, Victoria, Australia

REBECCA CHIBNALL, MD
Assistant Professor, Department of Dermatology, Washington University School of
Medicine, St Louis, Missouri, USA

GABRIELA A. COBOS, MD
Resident Physician, Ronald O. Perelman Department of Dermatology, NYU Langone
Dermatologic Associates, New York, New York, USA

RACHEL I. KORNIK, MD
Assistant Professor, Department of Dermatology, University of Wisconsin–Madison,
Madison, Wisconsin, USA

CATHERINE M. LECLAIR, MD
Professor of Obstetrics and Gynecology, Director, Program in Vulvar Health, Chief,
Division of General Obstetrics and Gynecology, Oregon Health & Science University,
Portland, Oregon, USA

MELISSA MAUSKAR, MD
Assistant Professor, Department of Dermatology, UT Southwestern Medical Center,
Dallas, Texas, USA

LYNNE H. MORRISON, MD
Associate Professor of Dermatology, Director, Dermatologic Immunopathology Lab, Oregon Health & Science University, Portland, Oregon, USA

RITA PICHARDO-GEISINGER, MD
Associate Professor, Department of Dermatology, Wake Forest School of Medicine, Winston-Salem, North Carolina, USA

MIRIAM KELTZ POMERANZ, MD
Associate Professor, Ronald O. Perelman Department of Dermatology, NYU Langone Dermatologic Associates, New York, New York, USA

STEPHANIE A. PRENDERGAST, MPT
Pelvic Health and Rehabilitation Center, Los Angeles, California, USA

JASON C. REUTTER, MD
Dermatopathologist, Piedmont Pathology Associates Inc, Hickory, North Carolina, USA

ALISON S. RUSTAGI, PhD
University of California, San Francisco School of Medicine, San Francisco, California, USA

AMY L. STENSON, MD, MSc
Associate Professor, Program in Vulvar Health, Department of Obstetrics and Gynecology, Oregon Health & Science University, Portland, Oregon, USA

KRISTEN M.A. STEWART, MD
Total Dermatology Care Center, Jacksonville, Florida, USA

ANUJA VYAS, MD, FACOG
Assistant Professor, Department of Obstetrics and Gynecology, Baylor College of Medicine, Houston, Texas, USA

Contents

The evaluation of the vulva should always begin with a detailed clinical history. The clinician should be very familiar with vulvar anatomy and the changes it undergoes depending on the patient's age and hormonal status. A systematic approach should be developed when examining the vulva so as to not leave out any parts. Finally, there is a wide array of ancillary tests and diagnostic procedures that can be pursued to arrive at the correct diagnosis and begin proper management.

Certain adjustable factors may influence how helpful a pathology report is to the clinician. Different biopsy techniques may be preferable based on the type of lesion being biopsied and the background epithelial surface. Key observations from the history and physical examination, possibly with a clinical photograph, are helpful to the pathologist. When reading the pathology report, the clinician should realize the difficulties arising from definitively classifying some diseases and how treatment can affect the tissue. Finally, miscommunication with the pathologist must be avoided by understanding the current nomenclature of vulvar disease.

Cutaneous vulvar neoplasms are commonly encountered at gynecology visits, with 2% of women having a benign vulvar melanocytic nevus and 10% to 12% of nevi being vulvar. High-grade squamous intraepithelial lesions (vulvar intraepithelial neoplasia 2 or 3) occur in 5 per 100,000 women, with an increasing incidence in the past 30 years. The recognition of these lesions and differentiation between benign, premalignant, and malignant stages are crucial for adequate diagnosis, clinical monitoring, and treatment. The presentation, diagnosis, and management of benign and malignant vulvar proliferations are discussed with focus on the practical aspects of clinical care.

Red patches and plaques of the vulva may be manifestations of neo-plasms, infections, or inflammatory skin diseases. These diseases can mimic one another clinically; features that generally allow the diseases to be identified on most cutaneous surfaces can be altered in the moist, occluded vulvar environment, making clinical diagnosis difficult. A detailed history and thorough physical examination can point to the likely diagnosis, but biopsy and culture may be needed for diagnosis especially in refractory disease. It is not uncommon for several of these processes to be present concomitantly or complicating other vulvar diseases.

Pruritus, or itch, is a common vulvar complaint that is often treated empir-ically as a yeast infection; however, yeast infections are just one of the many conditions that can cause vulvar itch. Ignoring other conditions can prolong pruritus unnecessarily. Atopic dermatitis, irritant contact dermatitis, and allergic contact dermatitis are extremely common noninfectious causes of vulvar itch that are often underdiagnosed by nondermatologists. Identifying these conditions and treating them appro-priately can significantly improve a patient's quality of life and appropri-ately decrease health care expenditures by preventing unnecessary additional referrals or follow-up visits and decreasing pharmaceutical costs.

Vulvar pruritus and lichen simplex chronicus are common reasons for presentation to women's health practitioners, including gynecologists and dermatologists. Both conditions are multifactorial and are often confounded by other inflammatory, neoplastic, infectious, environmental, neuropathic, hormonal, and behavioral variables. Careful history taking and thorough physical examinations, including wet mount and potentially skin biopsy, are necessary for appropriate diagnosis. Treatment should focus on decreasing inflammation, reducing irritants, and providing symp-tomatic relief to achieve remission. Comprehensive treatment covering environmental, biological, and behavioral therapy can result in long-term cure for patients with these conditions.

A variety of disorders may be confused with vulvar or genital lichen scle-rosus, as they can share several common features. This article dis-cusses the diagnosis, workup, and management of vulvar lichen sclerosus, with specific attention on distinguishing it from other derma-tologic mimics.

Lichen planus is an inflammatory mucocutaneous condition with a myriad of clinical manifestations. There are 3 forms of lichen planus that affect the vulva: papulosquamous, hypertrophic, and erosive. Erosive lichen planus can progress to vulvar scaring, vaginal stenosis, and squamous cell carcinoma; these long-term sequelae cause sexual distress, depression, and decreased quality of life for patients. Diagnosis is often delayed because of patient embarrassment or clinician misdiagnosis. Early recognition and treatment is essential to decreasing the morbidity of this condition. Multimodal treatment, along with a multidisciplinary approach, will improve outcomes and further clinical advances in studying this condition.

Vulvar fissures, excoriations, and erosions are common problems resulting from a variety of causes, many involving other mucosal and cutaneous sites. The authors present historical and examination features and useful investigations that can help establish a diagnosis so that definitive therapy can be instituted. Vulvar involvement also can be part of life-threatening conditions that require hospital admission and a multidisciplinary approach for optimal patient care. The clinical morphology of these examination findings and response to therapy can be modified by various host factors, particularly immune status, and atypical presentations and responses to therapy should always prompt patient reevaluation.

This article discusses the differential diagnosis of vulvar ulcers and describes a general clinical approach to this common but nonspecific examination finding. The differential diagnosis includes sexually and nonsexually transmitted infections, dermatitides, trauma, neoplasms, hormonally induced ulcers, and drug reactions. Patient history and physical examination provide important clues to the cause of a vulvar ulcer. However, laboratory testing is usually required for accurate diagnosis because the clinical presentation is often nonspecific and may be atypical due to secondary conditions.

This article discusses the clinical evaluation and approach to patients with 3 complex ulcerative vulvar conditions: hidradenitis suppurativa, metastatic Crohn disease of the vulva, and aphthous ulcers. These conditions are particularly challenging to medical providers because, although each is known to present with nonspecific examination findings that vary in morphology, the predominance of the diagnosis is based on clinical examination and exclusion of a wide variety of other conditions. Care of patients with these conditions is further complicated by the lack of therapeutic data and the significant impact these conditions have on quality of life.

Vulvovaginal chronic graft-versus-host disease (cGVHD) is an underrecognized complication of stem cell transplantation. Early recognition may prevent severe sequelae. Genital involvement is associated with oral, ocular, and skin manifestations. Treatment includes topical immunosuppression, dilator use, and adjuvant topical estrogen. Clinical and histologic features may mimic other inflammatory vulvar conditions. In the right clinical context, these findings are diagnostic of cGVHD. Female recipients of allo-hematopoietic stem cell transplantation (HCT) are at higher risk of condylomas, cervical dysplasia, and neoplasia. The National Institutes of Health publishes guidelines for the diagnosis, grading, management, and supportive care for HCT patients by organ system.

Vulvodynia is a common condition that negatively affects sexual health and quality of life for many women. A new classification system that divides vulvodynia into subtypes based on pain characteristics has been adopted. Diagnosis relies on ruling out possible contributing pathologic conditions. A multidisciplinary approach to treatment is likely to achieve the best outcome for all types. Medical therapy with systemic neuromodulators is suggested for generalized vulvodynia. For patients with vestibulodynia, topical therapy may be beneficial. Vestibulectomy has a high success rate and may be a good option if the patient is not responding to treatment.

Vulvar pain affects up to 20% of women at some point in their lives, and most women with vulvar pain have associated pelvic floor impairments. Pelvic floor dysfunction is associated with significant functional limitations in women by causing painful intercourse and urinary, bowel, and sexual dysfunction. A quick screening of the pelvic floor muscles can be performed in the gynecology office and should be used when patients report symptoms of pelvic pain. It is now known the vulvar pain syndromes are heterogeneous in origin; therefore, successful treatment plans are multimodal and include physical therapy.

OBSTETRICS AND GYNECOLOGY CLINICS

THE CLINICS ARE AVAILABLE ONLINE!
Access your subscription at:
www.theclinics.com

Foreword

Differentiating Between Normal, Benign, and Potentially Serious Vulvar Conditions

 CrossMark

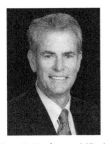

William F. Rayburn, MD, MBA
Consulting Editor

This issue of the *Obstetrics and Gynecology Clinics of North America*, edited by Aruna Venkatesan, MD, is dedicated to the diagnosis and management of vulvar disorders. This subject has not been discussed in past issues, and coverage has long been overdue. A wide spectrum of normal, benign, premalignant, and malignant lesions may occur on the vulva. For many physicians, patient symptoms require a rapid inspection and probably a prescription of medication and hygiene recommendations, with a follow-up as necessary. Furthermore, any vulvar conditions may be asymptomatic and, with fewer pelvic exams being performed routinely, there is more opportunity for any disorder to worsen.

The first article begins with the diagnostic evaluation of women with vulvar lesions. A history is obtained by asking questions relating to how long the lesion was present, when it first appeared, and any accompanying symptoms (eg, itching, burning, pain, discharge). Other questions relate to any lesions located orally, vaginally, or anally; accompanying incontinence; family history of similar vulvar disease; and skin care and hygiene routines. Prescription or over-the-counter medications, personal care products, and home remedies should be sought and any response to therapy.

Before physical examination, it would be prudent to have a female assistant in the room, sufficient lighting, any magnifying lens such as a colposcope, a mirror for the patient to identify the lesion, a ruler, and a camera. Any lesions should be recorded according to its size and shape, type (eg, macule, nodule, ulcer, plaque, pustule, cyst), edge, number and location, color, consistency and feel, and discomfort from inflammation. For completeness, other structures, such as the anus, vagina, cervix, regional lymph nodes, bruises or lacerations, and eye, mouth, and nares, should be examined routinely, since vulvar lesions may indicate a more widespread disease.

Obstet Gynecol Clin N Am 44 (2017) xi–xii
http://dx.doi.org/10.1016/j.ogc.2017.06.002
0889-8545/17/© 2017 Published by Elsevier Inc.

obgyn.theclinics.com

The diagnosis of many vulvar conditions is frequently clinical and does not require any procedures. However, a vaginal pH and wet mount may be helpful for patients with an accompanying vaginal discharge and evaluation of a sexually transmitted disease, especially if an ulceration is evident. Vulvar cytology is discouraged because of its poor correlation with tissue diagnosis. Lesions, especially on magnification, are to be biopsied when suspicious for malignancy, do not resolve after standard therapy, or cannot be diagnosed with confidence especially when accompanied by further patient concerns. A drawing or photograph of the lesion(s) is often helpful.

The second article pertaining to high-yield histopathology provides an excellent oversight about the range of vulvar disorders. The authors bring their expertise in describing the specific means for diagnosing and treating common conditions such as neoplasms, dermatitis, pruritic lesions, lichen sclerosus, erosive lichen planus, and erosive or ulcerative vulvar conditions. The article pertaining to vulvovaginal graft-versus-host disease provides much insight into an unusual condition. In contrast, vulvodynia is more common, which can be a source of frustration in diagnosis and especially management. The description of pelvic floor physical therapy is a practical overview.

This *Obstetrics and Gynecology Clinics of North America* issue should be an invaluable contribution to any obstetrician-gynecologist's library. It should serve as an excellent resource in the office setting. I appreciate Dr Venkatesan's effort in organizing this publication and in enlisting the cooperation of expert dermatologists, obstetrician-gynecologists, pathologists, and physical therapists who shared their experience in a balanced, evidence-based, and enlightening manner.

William F. Rayburn, MD, MBA
Obstetrics and Gynecology
Continuing Medical Education and
Professional Development
University of New Mexico School of Medicine
MSC 10 5580, 1 University of New Mexico
Albuquerque, NM 87131-0001, USA

E-mail address:
WRayburn@salud.unm.edu

Preface

Evaluation and Management of Vulvar Disease

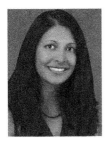

Aruna Venkatesan, MD, FAAD
Editor

In medicine there are certain groups of diseases that lie at the juncture between multiple specialties. Patients with these conditions often bounce from one provider to the next. Even the best providers may feel ill equipped to evaluate and manage these often difficult-to-diagnose and debilitating conditions. Vulvar disorders are one of these groups of diseases, and it is an honor as a dermatologist to guest edit this issue of *Obstetrics and Gynecology Clinics of North America* on the Evaluation and Management of Vulvar Disease.

Inevitably "orphan diseases" often provide the opportunity for rich interdisciplinary work. Vulvar disorders are no different. The authors highlighted in this issue illustrate this point well. They are nationally and internationally known dermatologists, obstetrician-gynecologists, pathologists, and physical therapists, all of whom have committed their careers to vulvar disorder management and education.

Each article in this issue was carefully selected for inclusion as a high-yield review of practical clinical tips for clinicians evaluating and managing patients with a vulvar chief complaint. The issue begins with an overview to managing vulvar disorders by Dr Gabriela Cobos and Dr Miriam Keltz Pomeranz. Dr Jason Reutter next reviews high-yield vulvar histopathology, which is critical for evaluating vulvar disorders. Dr Jill Allbritton then highlights important vulvar neoplasms. We then present an article structured around a common clinical presentation rather than a specific diagnosis—red rashes by Dr Lynne Morrison and Dr Catherine Leclair. Pruritic (itchy) vulvar rashes are subsequently highlighted by Dr Rita Pichardo-Geisinger (atopic and contact dermatitis) and Dr Rebecca Chibnall (vulvar pruritus and lichen simplex chronicus). We then move on to review two scarring vulvar dermatoses—genital lichen sclerosus and its mimics by Dr Anuja Vyas and erosive lichen planus by Dr Melissa Mauskar. The issue then transitions to conditions with varying degrees of epithelial disruption. Dr Tanja Bohl reviews a few specific erosive vulvar disorders. Dr Kristen Stewart provides a clinical approach

http://dx.doi.org/10.1016/j.ogc.2017.06.001
0889-8545/17/© 2017 Published by Elsevier Inc.
obgyn.theclinics.com

to vulvar ulcers and subsequently highlights a few specific challenging ulcerative vulvar conditions. Dr Rachel Kornik and Dr Alison Rustagi provide a welcome addition to the literature by reviewing vulvovaginal graft-versus-host-disease. Finally, the challenging condition vulvodynia is addressed through two articles. Dr Amy Stenson highlights its diagnosis and management, and pelvic floor physical therapist Stephanie Prendergast provides a clinician's guide to pelvic floor physical therapy.

I would like to especially thank Dr Libby Edwards and Dr Joanna Badger, two vulvology mentors, who have selflessly taught me all that I know about vulvar disease, and just as importantly, how to mentor budding vulvologists and give back to the field. I would not be where I am today without them, and I wouldn't be able to help the patients that I help without them.

It is a privilege to do this work alongside the mentors and colleagues mentioned above. After reading this issue, I hope you can see that the future of vulvology is bright.

Aruna Venkatesan, MD, FAAD
Division of Dermatology
Santa Clara Valley Medical Center
751 South Bascom Avenue, Suite 510
San Jose, CA 95128, USA

Department of Dermatology
Stanford University
Stanford, CA 94063, USA

E-mail address:
arunav@stanford.edu

A General Approach to the Evaluation and the Management of Vulvar Disorders

CrossMark

Gabriela A. Cobos, MD, Miriam Keltz Pomeranz, MD*

KEYWORDS

- Vulvar anatomy • Vulvar evaluation • Vulvar dermatology • Vulvar disorders

KEY POINTS

- A thorough clinical history and a systematic approach to the physical examination are paramount to the evaluation of vulvar disorders.
- The clinician must be aware of expected changes that the vulva undergoes depending on the patient's age and hormonal status.
- There are a wide variety of ancillary tests and diagnostic procedures available to help aid in diagnosis of vulvar disorders.

To begin the vulvar evaluation, the clinician must take a thorough clinical history, be familiar with the anatomy of the vulva and its normal variants, and appreciate that alterations of the vulva can occur depending on the patient's age and hormonal status.

CLINICAL HISTORY

As part of the clinical history, a detailed timeline is of utmost importance. Duration, progression (eg, constant, waxes, and wanes), severity, and any modifying factors (eg, occurs before menses, after intercourse, after grooming habits) should be elicited. The clinician should also establish whether the patient suffers from other skin conditions such as atopic dermatitis, psoriasis, or lichen planus. A detailed history regarding hygiene techniques should be acquired, focusing on the use of douches, chemical wipes, over-the-counter antibiotic ointments, antiseptics or topical analgesics, and the use of scrubbing instruments such as loofahs and washcloths.[1,2] A thorough sexual history is crucial. The use of contraceptives, lubricants, and toys should be elicited. It is also important to inquire about the patient's partner's product use because

Disclosure Statement: The authors have nothing to disclose.
Ronald O. Perelman Department of Dermatology, NYU Dermatologic Associates, 240 East 38th Street, 12th Floor, New York, NY 10016, USA
* Corresponding author.
E-mail address: Miriam.pomeranz@nyumc.org

Obstet Gynecol Clin N Am 44 (2017) 321–327
http://dx.doi.org/10.1016/j.ogc.2017.04.001
0889-8545/17/© 2017 Elsevier Inc. All rights reserved.

obgyn.theclinics.com

patients can develop an allergic contact dermatitis due to transfer of allergens from another person, referred to as consort or connubial dermatitis.[3]

ANATOMY

The vulva (**Fig. 1**) refers to the female external genitalia and is composed of the following mucocutaneous structures[2,4]:

1. Mons pubis is the anterior border of the vulva.
2. Genitocrural folds are the lateral borders.
3. Labia majora are covered with keratinized, hair-bearing skin on the lateral aspect, whereas the medial aspects are covered with partially keratinized skin, which contain subtle hair follicles.
4. Labia minora are covered with partially keratinized skin that contains subtle hair follicles. They also contain apocrine sweat glands and ectopic sebaceous glands, which are often most prominent on their medial aspect.
5. Clitoral hood or prepuce is formed by the fusion of the labia minora anteriorly. This structure should be retractable and covers the tip of the body of the clitoris. The body of the clitoris contains 2 corpora cavernosa, which are composed of erectile tissue.
6. Vestibule, which is also known as the introitus, is mucous membrane that extends from the medial aspect of the labia minora to the hymenal ring. The anterior and posterior borders are the clitoral frenulum and fourchette, respectively. It contains variable number of mucus-secreting glands, which supplement lubrication in young postpubertal women.
7. Bartholin glands are found in the posterior portion of vestibule at the 5 and 7 o'clock positions.
8. Skene glands are located lateral to the urethral meatus.

It should be noted that there is a paucity of data regarding what constitutes normal vulvar anatomy. More recently, there have been several papers, which showed that there is a wide range in measurements of different vulvar characteristics, such as

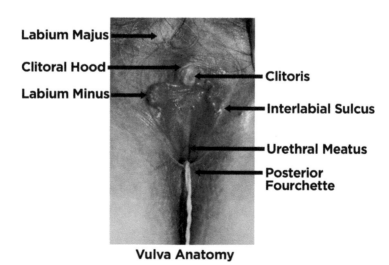

Vulva Anatomy

Fig. 1. Diagram of the vulva.

the length and width of the clitoris, labia minora, and labia majora, in both prepubertal girls and women.[5–11] Clinicians should keep this variability in mind before labeling certain anatomic features as abnormal.

As previously noted, the vulva undergoes changes depending on the woman's age and hormonal status. During childhood, the mons pubis and labia majora lose subcutaneous fat and the skin overlying these structures becomes thinner. Due to a lack of estrogen during childhood, the small labia minora may become adherent to each other. During puberty, due to increase in sex hormones, there is development of pubic hair, increase in dermal fat of the mons pubis and labia majora, and an increase in pigmentation of the vulva. The clitoris becomes more prominent and the cervix, vagina, labia minora, and vestibule increase in size. The vaginal fluid becomes acidic due to an increase in the intracellular concentration of glycogen and its metabolism by lactobacilli.[2,12–14] During pregnancy, further hyperpigmentation of the vulva may be observed. During menopause, decreased levels of estrogen can lead to changes in the pubic hair (more sparse and gray) and a decrease in subcutaneous fat of the labia majora and decrease in size of the labia minora. Vaginal epithelium becomes thin, pale, and dry due to a decrease in secretions. There is an increase in vaginal pH due to the decrease in intracellular glycogen stores, which results in a decrease of lactobacilli bacteria.[2,12–14]

EXAMINATION

Before beginning the examination, the patient should be instructed to completely remove her underwear to maximize exposure. If available, she should place her feet in stirrups. If there is no access to stirrups, then the patient should be supine and place her legs in a frog-leg position.[4] The clinician should develop a systematic, consistent approach for vulvar examination to make sure all parts are examined. The authors usually begin by assessing the mons pubis, assessing the hair distribution, the genitocrural folds, and inguinal folds. Next, we examine the clitoris and make sure the prepuce is easily retracted. We then assess the labia majora, labia minora, vestibule, perineum, and perianal area. While conducting the examination, there is attention to skin or mucosal color, texture, any lesions present, and anything else that seems unusual.[2]

In regard to color, the clinician should keep in mind that mild erythema or redness of the vulva and vagina is normal and can vary from patient to patient.[4,15] This erythema is usually more easily observed in patients of lighter complexion. If there is a deep or intense red color present, it can be concerning for hemorrhage, which can be seen in lichen sclerosus. It should also be noted that patients rarely examine their vulva when there is no pathologic abnormality present; thus, one should be cautious to attribute their symptoms to redness the patient has recently observed. Overall, color plays less of a vital role when assessing vulvar disorders compared with elsewhere on the body, with the exception of assessing a lesion that is suspicious for melanoma.

Texture should also be assessed because it can provide clues to the correct diagnosis. For example, in lichen sclerosus there is roughness due to slight hyperkeratosis. Lichenification refers to skin that is thickened and rough with an increase in skin markings. It is due to constant rubbing and points to chronic pruritic skin conditions such as atopic dermatitis.

The presence of primary lesions, such as macules, papules, or ulcers, should be noted. Clinicians need to become familiar with normal variants that can cause such lesions. For example, vulvar papillomatosis presents with fine, filiform papules, but their acuminate tips, discrete bases of adjacent lesions, and symmetric pattern help to distinguish them from condyloma acuminata.[4] Thus the morphology, location, and size of the lesion are crucial in forming a differential diagnosis, which will direct if further testing is needed; for guiding treatment; and for following for subsequent changes in the examination.

ANCILLARY TESTS

After detailed observation of the vulva is completed, the clinician can decide if additional tools are needed, such as speculum examination, vulvoscopy, or dermoscopy. A speculum examination can be performed to assess vaginal mucosa because there is often an overlap between vulvar and vaginal problems.[2] Vaginal discharge can be collected with cotton swabs for evaluation of pH and for further microscopic examination. To perform wet mount microscopy, the vaginal fluid collected is smeared onto 2 slides. A drop of normal saline is added to a slide while 1 drop of potassium hydroxide is added to the second slide. After placing a cover slip, the specimens are analyzed under the microscope. Wet mounts can be used to diagnose yeast, trichomonas, and bacterial vaginosis. Additionally, the maturity of epithelial cells can be assessed with a wet mount. Immature epithelial cells are rounder and smaller compared with mature epithelial cells but have proportionately larger nuclei. These immature epithelial cells can be a marker of estrogen-deficient vaginal epithelium but are also seen if there are erosions present or in rapidly proliferating epithelium.[4] Some clinicians calculate the vaginal maturation index (VMI) or the vaginal maturation value based on cytology to help assess for estrogen deficiency, and the VMI is commonly used in research protocols.[16]

Vulvoscopy, which is the use of a colposcope for examination of the vulva, remains controversial. Certain studies found its use beneficial for diagnosing premalignant lesions, but other studies did not find it effective as a screening tool and do not recommend its routine use.[2,17–21] Vulvoscopy can have a role in the examination of women with preinvasive disease. Of note, the use of stains such as acetic acid has been studied more objectively than the use of vulvoscopy itself.[19] Studies focusing on the use of 5% acetic acid as a predictor of subclinical human papillomavirus infection found its sensitivity was only 44%, specificity was 68%, and positive predictive value was 26%.[19,22] An advantage of an examination with a colposcope is that it provides optimal lighting and magnification without the need of close proximity between patient and provider.

The use of dermoscope, a handheld light source and magnifying device for evaluation of both pigmented and nonpigmented lesions is common practice among dermatologists. It allows for magnification and appreciation of structures in the epidermis and upper dermis that are not otherwise seen. When used by an experienced clinician, it allows for discernment of benignity of pigmented lesions and decreases unnecessary biopsies. It also aids in identification of certain infections and infestations such as molluscum contagiosum, pubic lice, and scabies.[4] The downside of dermoscopy is that it requires close proximity between the clinician and the lesion being examined. It also requires training as to what are benign structures and what are worrisome features.

The cotton swab test is a bedside test that is useful for evaluation of vulvodynia, which should be suspected when a patient complains of pain and/or burning without any findings on inspection of the vulva. The test is performed by placing the cotton swab at various vulvar locations. The clinician asks the patient to indicate where the light touch causes any discomfort, pain, itching, or burning. The test is useful to distinguish between localized or generalized pain, and can serve as an objective marker by asking the patient for a numerical value on the amount of discomfort they are experiencing at each location. It can then be tracked in subsequent visits and help guide therapy.[23] It can also have a positive psychological impact because it helps to validate that their pain is real.

DIAGNOSTIC PROCEDURES

Cultures should be taken if there is concern for an infection. If there appears to be impetiginization, demonstrated by honey colored crusting, infections due to staphylococcal and streptococcal species must be ruled out. Perianal streptococcal dermatitis caused by group A B-hemolytic *Streptococcus* is more often described in children and presents with symptomatic perianal erythema that can progress to vulvovaginitis. However, more recently, there have been reports of streptococcal infections causing refractory symptomatic perianal erythema in adults, which resolves with antibiotic therapy.[24,25] As such, cultures should be taken in patients with persistent, refractory perianal erythema. Other indications for cultures are intense pruritus or significant maceration.

Genital biopsies should be pursued if a definitive diagnosis is required and cannot be made clinically. There are a variety of different techniques, such as punch biopsy, shave biopsy, or snip excision with curved iris scissors, which is a variation of the shave biopsy. The depth of the pathologic abnormality should influence the choice of technique. For example, lichen sclerosus and lichen planus are fairly superficial dermal processes and pathologic abnormality could be adequately captured with a superficial biopsy. Therefore, in this setting, a shave biopsy or snip excision would be sufficient, though a superficial punch biopsy can also be done. However, if there is concern for deeper dermal or subcutaneous processes or depth of lesion is important, as in melanoma, then a punch biopsy should be pursued.

Regardless of biopsy technique, for anesthesia the authors use 0.5 to 1 mL of lidocaine 1% with epinephrine, injected with a 30-gauge needle. Before infiltrating the skin, we cleanse the area and circle the lesion with a sterile marking pen because the lesion can blanch and become difficult to find after introduction of the anesthetic.

For punch biopsies, if the defect is small, it can be left open and let to heal by secondary intention. Hemostasis can be achieved with aluminum chloride or Monsel solution (ferric subsulfate) or gelatin sponge (absorbable gelatin sponge). For larger defects in which closure is required, nonabsorbable nylon suture can be used on keratinized, hair-bearing skin. On mucosal surfaces, nonabsorbable silk suture is the gold standard given its ease of handling and lack of irritancy. However, the braided configuration of silk suture increases the risk of infection.[4] Other options are the use of absorbable sutures, such as polyglactin.[21]

The authors perform shave biopsies for exophytic lesions or superficial processes using a number 15 scalpel blade. Of note, gradle scissors can also be used for pedunculated lesions. For flat lesions, light scoring can be achieved with the tip of the blade and then, using forceps, an edge of the specimen can be lightly held and lifted while the tissue is obtained with the scalpel. A snip excision, which is a modification of the shave biopsy, can also be used for flat lesions. In this technique, any 5-0 or 6-0 suture is placed through the lesion. By pulling gently on the sutures, the lesion is tented upwards and the specimen is obtained with a curved iris scissor.[4] For both shave biopsies and snip excisions, hemostasis is obtained with aluminum chloride.

Aside from biopsy technique, the clinician should also be able to discern the biopsy site that will be most likely to capture the underlying pathologic abnormality. A guiding principle is to sample the most active part of the lesion. For example, in ulcers, the biopsy should be taken at the edge. For white atrophic patches, the center of the patch should be biopsied. For lesions with nodules, the nodular component should be sampled.

If histopathology results are consistent with a spongiotic dermatitis or contact dermatitis is on the differential, then patch testing can be pursued. It should be noted that a biopsy is not a prerequisite for patch testing because this can be a completely clinical diagnosis. Additionally, patch testing is not always necessary because a thorough clinical history can often help the clinician find the culprit factor. Before patch testing, all unnecessary products should be removed and patients should be encouraged to comply with gentle hygiene techniques, such as washing area with only water, avoiding any harsh soaps, and using white cotton underwear. If after these interventions, there continues to be a dermatitis or it recurs after treatment is halted, then the patient can be referred to a dermatologist for patch testing.

Due to the increased hydration and friction of vulvar skin, it is highly susceptible to irritant reactions.[26] It is commonly agreed on that the rate of allergic and irritant contact dermatitis in patients suffering from vulvar symptoms is high.[2] Studies report a wide range of positive patch tests, 16% to 78%, which is most likely due to the subject population that is tested.[27,28] The authors recommend the use of the North American Standard Series (NASS) because it is a more comprehensive panel compared with the ready to use thin-layer rapid use epicutaneous test (TRUE) test series. Positive test results should be examined in context of patient and partner's product use.

In summary, the evaluation of the vulva should always begin with a detailed clinical history. The clinician should be very familiar with vulvar anatomy and the changes it undergoes, depending on the patient's age and hormonal status. A systematic approach should be developed when examining the vulva so as to not leave out any parts. Finally, there is a wide array of ancillary tests and diagnostics procedures that can be pursued to arrive at the correct diagnosis and begin proper management.

REFERENCES

1. Mex GO. Prurito vulvar: determinación de las causas más frecuentes y su tratamiento. Ginecol Obstet Mex 2015;83:179–88.
2. Sacher BC. The normal vulva, vulvar examination, and evaluation tools. Clin Obstet Gynecol 2015;58(3):442–52.
3. McFadden J. Proxy contact dermatitis, or contact dermatitis by proxy (consort or connubial dermatitis). Patch testing tips. New York: Springer Berlin Heidelberg; 2014. p. 115–22.
4. Edwards L, Lynch PJ, editors. Genital dermatology atlas. Philadelphia: Lippincott Williams & Wilkins; 2010. p. 1–30.
5. Andrikopoulou M, Michala L, Creighton SM, et al. The normal vulva in medical textbooks. J Obstet Gynaecol 2013;33:648–50.
6. Howarth H, Sommer V, Jordan FM. Visual depictions of female genitalia differ depending on source. Med Humanit 2010;36:75–9.
7. Rouzier R, Louis-Sylvestre C, Paniel BJ, et al. Hypertrophy of labia minora: experience with 163 reductions. Am J Obstet Gynecol 2000;182:35–40.
8. Michala L, Koliantzaki S, Antsaklis A. Protruding labia minora: abnormal or just uncool? J Psychosom Obstet Gynaecol 2011;32:154–6.
9. Lloyd J, Crouch NS, Minto CL, et al. Female genital appearance: 'normality' unfolds. BJOG 2005;112:643–6.
10. Basaran M, Kosif R, Bayar U, et al. Characteristics of external genitalia in pre- and postmenopausal women. Climacteric 2008;11:416–21.

11. Akbiyik F, Kutlu AO. External genital proportions in prepubertal girls: a morphometric reference form female genotoplasty. J Urol 2010;184:1476–81.
12. Farage MA, Maibach HI. Morphology and physiological changes of genital skin and mucosa. Curr Probl Dermatol 2011;40:9–19.
13. Wingo C, Abdullatif H. Anatomy of female puberty: the clinical relevance of developmental changes in the reproductive system. Clin Anat 2013;26:115–29.
14. Neill SM, Lewis FM. Basics of vulval embryology, anatomy and physiology. In: Neill SM, Lewis FM, editors. Ridley's the vulva. 3rd edition. West Sussex (United Kingdom): Wiley-Blackwell; 2009. p. 1–33.
15. Van Beurden M, van der Vange N, de Craen AJ, et al. Normal findings in vulvar examination and vulvoscopy. Br J Obstet Gynaecol 1997;104:320–4.
16. Weber MA, Limpens J, Roovers JP. Assessment of vaginal atrophy: a review. Int Urogynecol J 2015;26(1):15–28.
17. Reid R, Greenberg MD, Daoud Y, et al. Colposcopic findings in women with vulvar pain syndromes. A preliminary report. J Reprod Med 1988;33:523–32.
18. MacLean AB, Reid WM. Benign and premalignant diseases of the vulva. Br J Obstet Gynaecol 1995;102:359–63.
19. Eva LI. Screening and follow up of vulval skin disorders. Best Pract Res Clin Obstet Gynaecol 2012;26:175–88.
20. Micheletti L, Bogliatto F, Lynch PJ. Vulvoscopy: review of a diagnostic approach requiring clarification. J Reprod Med 2008;53:179–82.
21. Gagné HM. Colposcopy of the vagina and vulva. Obstet Gynecol Clin North Am 2008;35(4):659–69.
22. Jonsson M, Karlson R, Evander M, et al. Acetowhitening of the cervix and vulva as a predictor of subclinical Human Papillomavirus infection: sensitivity and specificity in a population based study. Obstet Gynecol 1997;90:744–77.
23. Stockdale CK, Lawson HW. 2013 vulvodynia guideline update. J Low Genit Tract Dis 2014;18:93–100.
24. Kahlke V, Jongen J, Peleikis HG, et al. Perianal streptococcal dermatitis in adults: its association with pruritic anorectal diseases is mainly caused by group B Streptococci. Colorectal Dis 2013;15(5):602–7.
25. Neri I, Bardazzi F, Marzaduri S, et al. Perianal streptococcal dermatitis in adults. Br J Dermatol 1996;135(5):796–8.
26. Farage MA. Vulvar susceptibility to contact irritants and allergens: a review. Arch Gynecol Obstet 2005;272(2):167–72.
27. Bauer A, Oehme S, Geier J. Contact sensitization in the anal and genital area. Curr Probl Dermatol 2011;40:133–41.
28. Haverhoek E, Reid C, Gordon L, et al. Prospective study of patch testing in patients with vulval pruritus. Australas J Dermatol 2008;49:80–5.

High-Yield Vulvar Histopathology for the Clinician

Jason C. Reutter, MD

KEYWORDS

• Vulvar • Biopsy • Requisition • Pathology • Report • Diagnosis

KEY POINTS

- Where and how to biopsy is influenced by the lesion and location.
- An ideal requisition form contains a description of the lesion, differential diagnosis/clinical impression, and a photograph.
- When reading the report, be aware of instances of poor clinical pathologic correlation or alteration of histology caused by therapy and understand current terminology.

INTRODUCTION

It is an all too common scenario for a clinician to be frustrated by a pathology report that they receive. This is exacerbated by the patient's reluctance to agree to have the biopsy done in the first place. From the patient's perspective, they may be discouraged by previous unsuccessful empirical treatments or perhaps experience fear or embarrassment because of their condition. The clinician likewise may be vexed by their uncertainty and may have had difficulty procuring the biopsy because of the inherent challenges that arise from obtaining tissue from the genitalia.

This article offers tips to the clinician from the pathologist's perspective, which helps to increase the yield of obtaining useful information from biopsies. Focused attention on the nuances of performing the biopsy, filling out the requisition form (RF), and appraising the pathology report may maximize the information received by the clinician.

Disclosure Statement: The author has no relationships with any commercial company that has a direct financial interest in the subject matter or materials discussed in this article or with a company making a competing product.
Piedmont Pathology Associates, 1899 Tate Boulevard Southeast, Suite 1105, Hickory, NC 28601, USA
E-mail address: jasonreutter@gmail.com

PERFORMING BIOPSIES

The type of lesion and its general anatomic location should influence how the lesion is sampled and where precisely it is sampled. We will explore different instruments and techniques and other variables based on the lesion or type of epithelial surface.

Punch Biopsy

Punch biopsies are excellent tools for evaluating melanocytic lesions, ulcers, or any tumors or inflammatory processes with apparent deep involvement. In the case of melanocytic lesions, partial sampling of a melanoma is associated with misdiagnosis and microstaging inaccuracies.[1] Ideally one would completely excise a melanoma with narrow margins, which may be achieved with a punch instrument. When not feasible, one should attempt to get below the deepest portion of the tumor with the punch instrument because the single most important effector on the prognosis and treatment of melanoma is depth.[2] Shave saucerization specimens have yielded a 9% transection rate of melanoma, whereas punch specimens reduced the rate to 4% versus 1.5% with excisional specimens.[3]

Curved Iris Scissors

Sampling of modified mucous membranes (eg, labia minora) and mucous membranes (eg, introitus) may require a special technique. These moist surfaces may be difficult to grasp with instruments. Furthermore, the epithelium and subepithelium of mucosal surfaces do not adhere well when removed and may easily shear because of the lack of hair follicles to hold these structures together. This is particularly problematic in immunobullous disorders. Therefore, consideration of the technique of suture tenting with a curved iris scissors may be advisable in this situation (**Figs. 1** and **2**).[4]

Shave Biopsy

This technique is best reserved for hair-bearing, keratinized skin. Processes to consider for this method are superficial ones (eg, lichen sclerosus) and exophytic tumors (eg, fibroepithelial polyps).[4]

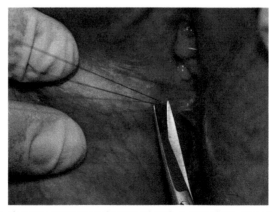

Fig. 1. Illustration of suture tenting and removal with a curved iris scissors. Minimal pressure is placed on the lesion, which is an erosive one based on mucous membranes. (*Courtesy of* L. Edwards, MD, Charlotte, NC.)

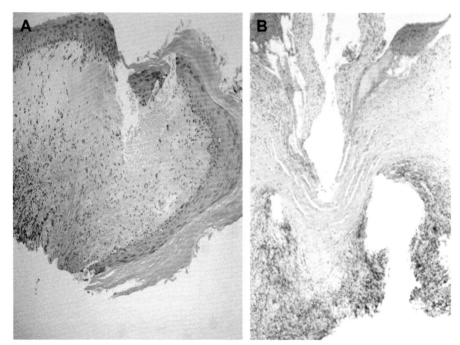

Fig. 2. Hematoxylin and eosin (original magnification ×100). Comparison of how the biopsy obtained with suture tenting (*A*) only leaves a small divot. No tissue is crushed. Compare this with (*B*) in which large divots are created with forceps and the intervening tissue is crushed and blurred.

Kevorkian Biopsy

Gynecologists typically have this instrument readily available and may choose to use it for vaginal biopsies. However, there is less precise manipulation of this device when targeting an area to biopsy.[4]

Specific Considerations Based on Type of Lesion

Ulcers
The highest yield of an ulcer is at the edge where the ulcer bed abuts intact epithelium. Biopsying the ulcer base may only yield necrotic tissue, and such diseases as herpes may be best visualized at the ulcer edge.

Lichen planus
Areas of mucosal lichen planus (LP) containing Wickham striae clinically may have a better chance of yielding more diagnostic features histologically.[5] Zegarelli[5] has recommended for biopsies of LP involving mucosal surfaces to attempt to capture Wickham striae in the specimen in a manner that could be captured histologically in multiple sections through the specimen (**Fig. 3**).

Immunobullous disorders
In general, lesional biopsies for routine histopathologic evaluation of mucosal immunobullous disorders should be obtained by a broad, long technique rather than a narrow deep biopsy to ensure tissue intactness.[6] Obtaining a perilesional specimen for direct immunofluorescence studies (DIF) is also necessary. A distance of 10 mm or

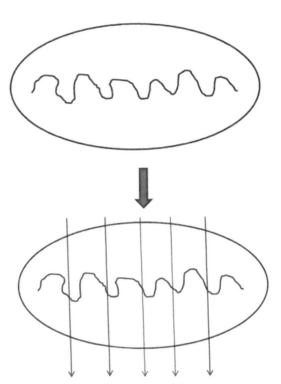

Fig. 3. Hypothetical Wickham striae in mucosal lichen planus are represented by the squiggly line and excised along the long axis by an elliptical specimen. The red lines represent cross-sectioning of the specimen by the laboratory, which captures the striae in each cross-section submitted for histology. (*Adapted from* Zegarelli DJ. Lichen planus: a simple and reliable biopsy technique. J Oral Med 1981;36(1):19; with permission.)

greater from the lesion for the DIF sample may ensure intactness of the tissue without sacrificing sensitivity.[7] Avoiding oral steroids for a month before the biopsy may also reduce the chance of a false-negative effect on immunoreactants.[8]

Avoiding Artifacts from Tissue Manipulation

One should not underestimate the permanent tissue damage that may be caused by forceps. It should be recognized that not only do forceps cause divots in tissue, but they permanently crush tissue in a distorted state in which cytologic detail is lost, particularly for lymphocytes (see **Fig. 2**).[9] Suture tenting, as described previously, may be a reasonable alternative.[4] Furthermore, using a needle to lift the tissue from a punch biopsy also may reduce the direct pressure on tissue.[4]

Fixation

The preferred media for fixation is buffered 10% formalin, with a volume of media 10 to 20 times the amount of the specimen.[9] With this fixation nearly any study including routine light microscopy, immunohistochemistry, and molecular studies can be performed. The only exceptions are specimens for DIF, which should be placed in Zeus or Michel media and material for cultures placed in a sterile container.

FILLING OUT THE REQUISITION FORM

The clinician should never underestimate the impact of carefully filling out an RF. Much has been written about critical information for the pathologist in the RF[10–14] and suggestions are present in **Box 1**. A belief that clinical information could bias the pathologist or that the diagnosis should be obvious on histology alone should be avoided.[13] Diagnoses may be made by synthesizing the clinical history, physical examination, and laboratory and histopathologic findings. For example, it was demonstrated in a Delphi consensus exercise among experts in vulvar disease that a diagnosis of erosive LP may be made by any combination of at least three of six different clinical findings and three different histopathologic findings.[15]

Although the RF commonly contains location and clinical impression, the morphology of the lesion, symptoms, and previous diagnoses are often excluded.[10] In general, particular points of interest include the distribution of lesions, because LP,[16] pemphigus,[17] mucous membrane pemphigoid,[18] and psoriasis[19] often have extravulvar involvement. Therefore, knowledge of lesions in other parts of the body is helpful to the pathologist. Knowledge of symptoms can also be a criterion in arriving at a diagnosis of erosive LP.[15] The size of the lesion, particularly in neoplasms, both epithelial and melanocytic, may guide the pathologist in determining their biologic significance. Nonetheless, of paramount importance is the appearance of the lesion. This includes such observations as erythema versus whitening versus pigmentation. If the pathologist is distracted by pigmentation and they are unaware that this is a normal baseline color for the patient's skin type, they may erroneously make a diagnosis of melanosis when that is not what the clinician is observing. Because of a distortion artifact that is commonly seen in the elastic skin of the vulva, many specimens round up and may be misinterpreted as fibroepithelial polyps. Therefore, it is important for the clinician to let the pathologist know whether this is a flattened lesion or polypoidal clinically.

In the case of clinical and pathologic discordance, an additional measure the pathologist may perform is deeper serial sections into the paraffin-embedded tissue block. These additional sections have been shown to produce an alternative impression in approximately 9% of skin samples.[20]

Clinical photographs are often not included in the RF,[10] but are believed to be helpful by dermatopathologists, particularly in inflammatory lesions.[21] Although this may be readily available to pathologists who work in the same institution as the clinician,

---

Box 1
Recommendations for items to consider on or with a requisition form for vulvar biopsies

- What the patient can tell you or what you can see
  - Distribution (including extravulvar)
  - Size of lesions
  - Appearance
    - Erythema
    - Ulcer
    - Skin-colored nodule
    - Pigmentation

- Description of what part of lesion biopsy was taken (eg, ulcer edge, white part of lesion, edge of blister)

- Clinical impression/differential diagnosis

- Photograph

it is wise for the clinician to consider sending encrypted clinical photographs via email, printing them out and attaching to the RF, sending via flash drive, or allowing to be accessed on a secure site.[21] The clinician may even consider in these photographs to ensure that inked areas indicate where the biopsy will be performed, or postbiopsy photographs may also let the pathologist know exactly where the sample has been taken.

Table 1
Common histologic findings used in the evaluation of inflammatory diseases of the vulva

Histologic Pattern	Definition	Possible Disease Implications
Spongiosis	Intercellular edema in the epithelium	• Irritant contact dermatitis • Allergic contact dermatitis • Atopic dermatitis (eczema) • Seborrheic dermatitis
Acanthosis	Thickening of the epithelium Subtypes include psoriasiform and verruciform	• Lichen simplex chronicus (either as a primary disease or secondary to other diseases) • Psoriasis • Rare neoplasms, such as differentiated vulvar intraepithelial neoplasia, may mimic these changes
Lichenoid	A band-like infiltrate of lymphocytes along the undersurface of the epithelium	• Lichen sclerosus • Lichen planus • Zoon vulvitis/plasma cell vulvitis (should contain plasma cells)
Homogenization/ hyalinization/ sclerosis	A glassy pink smudged alteration of the collagen	• Lichen sclerosus • Radiation dermatitis
Vesicle	Blister-like space	Subepithelial vesicles • Mucous membrane pemphigoid (cicatricial pemphigoid) • Linear IgA disease • Bullous pemphigoid
Acantholysis	Keratinocytes detach from one another in the epithelium losing their spinous processes	• Hailey-Hailey disease • Darier disease • Papular genitocrural acantholysis • Pemphigus • Herpes simplex virus
Granulomas	Large collections of histiocytes	• Crohn disease • Melkersson-Rosenthal syndrome • Infection • Foreign material
Vasculitis	Inflammation of vessels, particularly by neutrophils (leukocytoclastic vasculitis)	• Common causes of systemic vasculitis (eg, drug, infection, connective tissue disease) • Behçet syndrome • Nonspecific change underneath ulcer

Modified from Lynch PJ, Moyal-Barracco M, Bogliatto F, et al. 2006 ISSVD classification of vulvar dermatoses: pathologic subsets and their clinical correlates. J Reprod Med 2007;52(1):3–9; with permission.

In the era of electronic health records it is not too uncommon for pathologists to receive the clinical information in an RF populated with the correlating International Classification of Diseases-10 code. In these instances, the clinician should consider editing this with additional clinical data, particularly if the code does not indicate a specific diagnosis.

READING THE PATHOLOGY REPORT

The last phase, the postanalytical phase, is an equally important step for the clinician. In this phase, clinicians need to realize potential limitations to tissue evaluation.

Recognizing Potential Poor Clinical and Histopathologic Correlation

There is a poor correlation between duration of symptoms and the degree of development of histopathologic findings of lichen sclerosus.[22] Early developing histologic changes of LS are also difficult to separate from such diseases as LP and lichen simplex chronicus.[23,24] Genital or inverse psoriasis may not demonstrate the well-developed pathologic features of psoriasis that may be seen in other cutaneous sites and also may have additional features, such as spongiotic change, which could be

Table 2
Squamous intraepithelial neoplasia of the vulva as categorized by the ISSVD 2015 terminology

ISSVD 2015 Terminology	Significance	Alias Terminology
Low-grade squamous intraepithelial lesion of the vulva	Infection usually by low-risk HPV types causing viral cytopathic effect Using this term to describe atypia in less than or equal to the lower one-third of the vulvar epithelium without viral cytopathic effect, however, is discouraged because of the low reproducibility of this observation	Flat condyloma Condyloma accuminatum VIN 1 Mild dysplasia
High-grade squamous intraepithelial lesion of the vulva	Premalignant change in more than one-third of the epithelium often with a basaloid or warty appearance of the lesion Signifies involvement by high-risk HPV and diagnosis can often be supported by p16 block-like positivity as previously defined[31]	Usual VIN Classic VIN VIN 2 or VIN 3 Moderate or severe dysplasia Intraepithelial carcinoma, Bowen type
Differentiated VIN	Premalignant change often associated with an inflammatory dermatosis (eg, lichen sclerosus) rather than HPV Difficult to diagnose because of subtle histology Considered more aggressive than high-grade squamous intraepithelial lesions	Simplex-type VIN Intraepithelial carcinoma, simplex type Squamous cell hyperplasia with atypia

Abbreviations: HPV, human papilloma virus; VIN, vulvar intraepithelial neoplasia.
    Data from Bornstein J, Bogliatto F, Haefner HK, et al. The 2015 International Society for the Study of Vulvovaginal Disease (ISSVD) terminology of vulvar squamous intraepithelial lesions. Obstet Gynecol 2016;127(2):264–8.

misleading to the pathologist.[25] LP on genital skin, particularly mucosal surfaces, also has less pronounced findings than counterpart lesions elsewhere.[5,15,26]

Considering Effect of Previous Treatment

A markedly inflamed lesion clinically likely has marked inflammation histopathologically. Therefore, when lesions are partially treated, some of this inflammation may subside. However, common treatments, such as anesthetics, antibiotics, antifungals, and corticosteroids, may elicit an allergic contact dermatitis[27] that may add additional histopathologic features and perhaps an unusual clinical morphology. EMLA cream may also elicit nonspecific and unusual histopathologic changes.[28]

Use Current Terminology

A clinician is well served by keeping current on the terminology of vulvar diseases. An explanation of common histologic vernacular in the evaluation of vulvar inflammatory diseases as initially constructed by Lynch and colleagues[29] is presented in **Table 1**. The most recent development in terminology is in squamous intraepithelial neoplasia of vulva (**Table 2**). The International Society for the Study of Vulvovaginal Disease in 2015 markedly differed from the previous change in terminology of 2004.[30] Specifically, in parallel with the lower anogential squamous terminology,[31] the terms low-grade squamous intraepithelial lesion and high-grade squamous intraepithelial lesion are used for human papilloma virus–related lesions. However, the type of squamous neoplasia not associated with human papilloma virus is termed differentiated vulvar intraepithelial neoplasia. Compared with high-grade squamous intraepithelial lesion, differentiated vulvar intraepithelial neoplasia has a higher likelihood of developing[32] and shorter period of progressing into[33] invasive squamous cell carcinoma.

SUMMARY

The pathology report should be a helpful tool in the clinician's armamentarium in evaluating vulvar disease. Appropriately performed biopsies coupled with informative clinical data, an understanding of the limitations of vulvar tissue evaluation, and of current terminology can only increase its effectiveness.

REFERENCES

1. Ng JC, Swain S, Dowling JP, et al. The impact of partial biopsy on histopathologic diagnosis of cutaneous melanoma: experience of an Australian tertiary referral service. Arch Dermatol 2010;146(3):234–9.
2. Balch CM, Soong SJ, Atkins MB, et al. An evidence-based staging system for cutaneous melanoma. CA Cancer J Clin 2004;54(3):131–49.
3. Mir M, Chan CS, Khan F, et al. The rate of melanoma transection with various biopsy techniques and the influence of tumor transection on patient survival. J Am Acad Dermatol 2013;68(3):452–8.
4. Edwards L. Diagnostic and therapeutic techniques. In: Edwards L, Lynch PJ, editors. Genital dermatology atlas. 2nd edition. Philadelphia: Wolters Kluwer Health Lippincott Williams and Wilkins; 2011. p. 26–8.
5. Zegarelli DJ. Lichen planus: a simple and reliable biopsy technique. J Oral Med 1981;36(1):18–20.
6. Kumaraswamy KL, Vidhya M, Rao PK, et al. Oral biopsy: oral pathologist's perspective. J Cancer Res Ther 2012;8(2):192–8.

7. Sano SM, Quarracino MC, Aguas SC, et al. Sensitivity of direct immunofluorescence in oral diseases. Study of 125 cases. Med Oral Patol Oral Cir Bucal 2008;13(5):E287–91.
8. Jordan RC, Daniels TE, Greenspan JS, et al. Advanced diagnostic methods in oral and maxillofacial pathology. Part II: immunohistochemical and immunofluorescent methods. Oral Surg Oral Med Oral Pathol Oral Radiol Endod 2002; 93(1):56–74.
9. High WA, Tomasini CF, Argenziano G, et al. Basic prinicples of dermatology. In: Bolognia JL, Jorizzo JL, Schaffer JV, editors. Dermatology. 3rd edition. Elsevier Saunders; 2012. p. 12–6.
10. Olson MA, Lohse CM, Comfere NI. Rates of provision of clinical information in the skin biopsy requisition form and corresponding encounter visit note. J Pathol Inform 2016;7:40.
11. Wong C, Peters M, Tilburt J, et al. Dermatopathologists' opinions about the quality of clinical information in the skin biopsy requisition form and the skin biopsy care process: a semiqualitative assessment. Am J Clin Pathol 2015;143(4):593–7.
12. Comfere NI, Peters MS, Jenkins S, et al. Dermatopathologists' concerns and challenges with clinical information in the skin biopsy requisition form: a mixed-methods study. J Cutan Pathol 2015;42(5):333–45.
13. Chismar LA, Umanoff N, Murphy B, et al. The dermatopathology requisition form: attitudes and practices of dermatologists. J Am Acad Dermatol 2015;72(2): 353–5.
14. Waller JM, Zedek DC. How informative are dermatopathology requisition forms completed by dermatologists? a review of the clinical information provided for 100 consecutive melanocytic lesions. J Am Acad Dermatol 2010;62(2):257–61.
15. Simpson RC, Thomas KS, Leighton P, et al. Diagnostic criteria for erosive lichen planus affecting the vulva: an international electronic-Delphi consensus exercise. Br J Dermatol 2013;169(2):337–43.
16. Lewis FM, Shah M, Harrington CI. Vulval involvement in lichen planus: a study of 37 women. Br J Dermatol 1996;135(1):89–91.
17. Lim HW, Bystryn JC. Evaluation and management of diseases of the vulva: bullous diseases. Clin Obstet Gynecol 1978;21(4):1007–22.
18. Eschle-Meniconi ME, Ahmad SR, Foster CS. Mucous membrane pemphigoid: an update. Curr Opin Ophthalmol 2005;16(5):303–7.
19. Edwards L. Pediatric genital disease. In: Edwards L, Lynch PJ, editors. Genital dermatology atlas. 2nd edition. Philadelphia: Wolters Kluwer Health Lippincott Williams and Wilkins; 2011. p. 254.
20. Stuart LN, Rodriguez AS, Gardner JM, et al. Utility of additional tissue sections in dermatopathology: diagnostic, clinical and financial implications. J Cutan Pathol 2014;41(2):81–7.
21. Mohr MR, Indika SH, Hood AF. The utility of clinical photographs in dermatopathologic diagnosis: a survey study. Arch Dermatol 2010;146(11):1307–8.
22. Marren P, Millard PR, Wojnarowska F. Vulval lichen sclerosus: lack of correlation between duration of clinical symptoms and histological appearances. J Eur Acad Venerology Dermatol 1997;8:202–16.
23. Fung MA, LeBoit PE. Light microscopic criteria for the diagnosis of early vulvar lichen sclerosus: a comparison with lichen planus. Am J Surg Pathol 1998;22: 473–8.
24. Weyers W. Hypertrophic lichen sclerosus sine sclerosis: clues to histopathologic diagnosis when presenting as psoriasiform lichenoid dermatitis. J Cutan Pathol 2015;42(2):118–29.

25. Patterson JW. The psoriasiform reaction pattern. In: Patterson J, editor. Weedon's skin pathology. 4th edition. Chruchill Livingstone Elsevier; 2016. p. 89.

26. Luzar B, Calonje E. Noninfectious dermatoses of the vulva. In: Singh N, McCluggage WG, editors. Pathology of the vulva and vagina. London: Springer; 2013. p. 61.

27. Schlosser BJ. Contact dermatitis of the vulva. Dermatol Clin 2010;28(4):697–706.

28. Lewis FM, Agarwal A, Neill SM, et al. The spectrum of histopathologic patterns secondary to the topical application of EMLA® on vulvar epithelium: clinicopathological correlation in three cases. J Cutan Pathol 2013;40(8):708–13.

29. Lynch PJ, Moyal-Barracco M, Bogliatto F, et al. 2006 ISSVD classification of vulvar dermatoses: pathologic subsets and their clinical correlates. J Reprod Med 2007; 52(1):3–9.

30. Bornstein J, Bogliatto F, Haefner HK, et al, ISSVD Terminology Committee. The 2015 International Society for the Study of Vulvovaginal Disease (ISSVD) terminology of vulvar squamous intraepithelial lesions. J Low Genit Tract Dis 2016;20(1): 11–4.

31. Darragh TM, Colgan TJ, Cox JT, et al. The lower anogenital squamous terminology standardization project for HPV-associated lesions: background and consensus recommendations from the College of American Pathologists and the American Society for Colposcopy and Cervical Pathology. J Low Genit Tract Dis 2012;16(3):205–42.

32. Eva LJ, Ganesan R, Chan KK, et al. Differentiated-type vulval intraepithelial neoplasia has a high-risk association with vulval squamous cell carcinoma. Int J Gynecol Cancer 2009;19(4):741–4.

33. van de Nieuwenhof HP, Massuger LF, van der Avoort IA, et al. Vulvar squamous cell carcinoma development after diagnosis of VIN increases with age. Eur J Cancer 2009;45(5):851–6.

Vulvar Neoplasms, Benign and Malignant

Jill I. Allbritton, MD[a,b,c],*

KEYWORDS

- Melanosis • Genital nevi • Differentiated vulvar intraepithelial neoplasia (dVIN)
- High-grade squamous intraepithelial lesion (HSIL) • Squamous cell carcinoma (SCC)
- Basal cell carcinoma • Vulvar melanoma • Paget disease

KEY POINTS

- Many pigmented vulvar lesions are indistinguishable clinically and so require biopsy to evaluate for early melanoma.
- Simple excision is curative for dysplastic nevi and atypical nevi of the genital type.
- High-grade squamous intraepithelial lesions (HSIL; formerly vulvar intraepithelial neoplasia [VIN] 2 or 3) can be treated conservatively with imiquimod. Nonresponsive lesions need biopsy to evaluate for occult invasion.
- Differentiated VIN (dVIN) is often missed clinically and histologically. Although only accounting for 5% of vulvar dysplasia diagnoses, dVIN has a higher rate of progression to squamous cell carcinoma (SCC), shorter time interval to progression, and higher recurrence rate than HSIL.
- Prognosis of vulvar SCC correlates with lymph node invasion, size of tumor, and depth of stromal invasion.

VULVAR PIGMENTED LESIONS

Melanoma comprises 10% of vulvar pigmented lesions and occurs in the sixth to seventh decade.[1–3] The clinical goal of evaluating vulvar pigmented lesions is focused on eliminating the possibility of melanoma, which can be clinically indistinguishable from other pigmented lesions.[4]

BENIGN PIGMENTED VULVAR LESIONS

Vulvar melanoma is detected late, with a resulting poor prognosis of less than 50% 5-year survival. Detecting cutaneous melanoma early is a key component to

Disclosure Statement: The author has no conflicts of interest to disclose.
[a] Bethesda Dermpath Laboratory, 1730 Elton Road, Suite 11, Silver Spring, MD 20903, USA;
[b] Anne Arundel Dermatology, Towson, MD 21204, USA; [c] Pathology, Johns Hopkins University, 4940 Bayview Medical Center, Eastern Avenue, Baltimore, MD 21224, USA
* Bethesda Dermpath Laboratory, 1730 Elton Road, Suite 11, Silver Spring, MD 20903.
E-mail address: jilgardens@gmail.com

Obstet Gynecol Clin N Am 44 (2017) 339–352
http://dx.doi.org/10.1016/j.ogc.2017.04.002
0889-8545/17/© 2017 Elsevier Inc. All rights reserved.
obgyn.theclinics.com

reducing melanoma mortality.[5] From 10% to 12% of all cutaneous pigmented lesions occur on genital skin.[2] Vulvar compound and junctional nevi are the most common pigmented lesions of the vulva, comprising 55% of pigmented vulvar lesions. Percentages of pigmented vulvar lesions are summarized in **Table 1**. The small size (5 mm or less) and uniform pigmentation distinguish common nevi from melanoma. Change in an otherwise typical nevus or a nevus that appears different from the patient's other nevi, the so-called ugly-duckling sign, warrant a biopsy. Stable nevi should be followed clinically and do not require treatment.

MELANOTIC MACULES

Melanotic macules are common benign pigmented lesions located on labia minora, usually restricted to nonkeratinized skin in adult women. Melanotic macules make up 17% of vulvar pigmented lesions, and most are uniformly pigmented and of small size. If a pigmented lesion appears consistent with melanotic macule but is larger than 6 mm, biopsy should be considered because it is impossible to distinguish larger melanotic macules (>6 mm) from early vulvar melanoma. Multiple melanotic macules are seen in genetic syndromes, such as LAMB (lentigines, atrial myxoma, mucocutaneous myxomas, blue

Table 1
Percentages of pigmented vulvar lesions

Vulvar Pigmented Lesions	Percentage	Average Age (y)	Clinical Appearance	Treatment
Common nevi	55	34	1–5 mm, flesh colored, tan to dark brown, flat to dome shaped	Not indicated unless concern for melanoma exists
Melanotic macule (lentigo)	17	43	5 mm–2 cm tan to dark brown to black, flat, without elevation	Not indicated unless concern for melanoma exists
Melanoma	10	>55	Erythematous to black, solitary to multifocal, usually 6 mm or greater	Excision, staging per TNM protocol
Atypical nevus of genital type	10	21	6 mm or larger, erythematous to tan to black, may be asymmetric	Conservative excision
Dysplastic nevus	5	32	6 mm or larger, erythematous to tan to black, may be asymmetric	Conservative excision
Blue nevus	Rare	Unknown	5 mm or smaller, dark blue to black, flat to dome shaped	Not indicated unless concern for melanoma exists
Recurrent nevi	Rare	Unknown	Size varies, asymmetric color, size, irregular shape	Conservative excision
Vulvar melanosis	Rare	Unknown	Flat, asymmetric, tan to blue to black, irregular borders and size	Baseline photos, biopsy, clinical follow-up

Abbreviation: TNM, tumor, node, metastasis.

nevi), Peutz-Jeghers, LEOPARD (lentigines, electrocardiogram abnormalities, ocular hypertelorism, pulmonary stenosis, abnormalities of genitalia, retardation of growth, and deafness), Ruvalcaba-Myhre, and Laugier-Hunziker.[6] Children with multiple melanotic macules should be referred for genetic evaluation to exclude these syndromes.

VULVAR MELANOSIS

Unlike common nevi and melanotic macules, vulvar melanosis is a rare pigmented lesion, often multifocal, asymmetric, and irregularly pigmented. Vulvar melanosis most often arises on the labia minora but can occur on other nonkeratinized genital skin. The cause is unknown, hypothesized to be postinflammatory, and it is most commonly seen in women with lichen sclerosus (LS). Vulvar melanosis is clinically similar to early vulvar melanoma; both are variably pigmented, asymmetric, and can be multifocal. However, vulvar melanosis is seen in younger women than vulvar melanoma. Rare cases of vulvar melanoma are reported in young women. Therefore, photographic documentation, biopsy, and clinical follow-up are recommended. Large lesions (>1 cm) need multiple biopsy samples to adequately assess the underlying histology. Although vulvar melanosis is clinically indistinguishable from vulvar melanoma, vulvar melanosis carries no increased risk of melanoma development.[4,7]

DYSPLASTIC NEVI AND ATYPICAL NEVI OF THE GENITAL TYPE

Dysplastic nevi are considered markers of an increased risk of cutaneous melanoma rather than individual dysplastic nevi representing a premalignant lesion.[8] Only 6% of vulvar melanomas arise in nevi, in contrast with 33% of nongenital melanomas arising in preexisting nevi. Genital dysplastic nevi are most commonly located on hair-bearing genital skin. These lesions are typically 6 mm or greater with a dome-shaped erythematous to tan center and hyperpigmented more macular periphery, although many morphologies are possible. These lesions can be followed clinically if other similar atypical nevi are present and the lesion is stable in size and morphology.[4] A biopsy is necessary if the lesion has changed, the history of the lesion is in doubt, or the nevus looks clinically different from the patient's other nevi. Atypical nevi of the genital type (ATNGT) may be clinically indistinguishable from common nevi or dysplastic nevi, although they are typically larger than common nevi. These nevi are unique to genital sites and do not confer an increased risk of cutaneous melanoma, nor are they premalignant. They occur anywhere along the embryonic milk line, and are more common in women than in men.[4] Up to a third of these proliferations are histologically misdiagnosed as melanoma because they share some histologic features with melanoma, such as cytologic atypia, expansile junctional nests that may be dyscohesive, confluent basal melanocyte growth, and central upward migration of melanocytes (pagetoid growth). Although in ATNGT the cytologic atypia is uniform, the proliferation is symmetric with sharp lateral circumscription, and pagetoid growth is limited to the center of the proliferation. Simple excision is curative.[2]

RECURRENT NEVI

Recurrent nevus is a histologic diagnosis occurring on the vulva in patients with lichen sclerosis. The recurrent nevi are clinically atypical, with irregular borders and pigment distribution, and not associated with an evident scar. The background of fibrosis and dermal homogenization caused by lichen sclerosis causes the nevus to appear atypical clinically and histologically. Recurrent nevi share histologic features with melanoma, including upward migration of melanocytes into the superficial epidermis, dermal fibrosis, and enlarged melanocytes with ample cytoplasm containing granular melanin pigment.[9]

Recurrent nevi associated with lichen sclerosis can be distinguished from melanoma by the homogenization of the papillary dermis rather than the regression-associated fibrosis in melanoma. In recurrent nevi, pagetoid growth is limited to the epidermis overlying the dermal fibrosis. However, histologic distinction is difficult if a history of LS is not disclosed to the pathologist. These nevi require simple excision because of the color variation and asymmetry. The clinical history of LS needs to accompany the specimen so the correct pathologic diagnosis is reached.

MALIGNANT LIGMENTED VULVAR LESIONS
Melanoma

Ten percent of pigmented vulvar lesions are melanomas, most often occurring in the sixth to seventh decade, on the clitoris or labia minora. Up to 25% of vulvar melanomas are amelanotic, making clinical diagnosis more difficult.[4] The highest incidence of genital melanoma occurs in white women; this is different from other cutaneous melanomas, with the highest incidence in white men. Increasing age, advanced stage, and female sex correlate with decreased survival. Unlike the incidence of cutaneous melanoma which increased from 1982 to 2011, the incidence of vulvar melanoma remained stable from 1992 to 2012.[10] Distinctly different from other cutaneous melanomas, vulvar melanomas may be multifocal and more often arise de novo rather than in a preexisting nevus.[7] In addition, 28% of genital melanomas contain c-kit mutations, and 28% contain neuroblastoma RAS oncogene (NRAS) mutations, unlike melanomas that arise on intermittently ultraviolet light exposed skin, in which 40% to 50% contain B-raf proto-oncogene (BRAF) mutations.[5] Vulvar melanomas are detected late, with a mean size 30 mm, which leads to poor prognosis as determined by Breslow depth.[11] A Dutch study found a median Breslow depth of 4 mm for vulvar melanoma.[12]

DIAGNOSIS

Any new pigmented lesion in a postmenopausal woman; or a pigmented lesion with irregular size, color, or shape; or one that looks different from other cutaneous pigmented lesions requires biopsy. Because 25% of melanomas are nonpigmented, new or nonresolving erythematous papules and plaques require biopsy. In large lesions that cannot be completely sampled, multifocal sampling is recommended because histologic changes may vary within the lesion. Often a lentigo or benign nevus is present adjacent to melanoma in large pigmented lesions. The melanoma may be missed if the pigmented lesion is not adequately sampled. Because melanoma can be multifocal on genital sites, sampling of all irregularly shaped, asymmetric, or new pigmented lesions is advisable. Stable pigmented lesions can be followed with photographic documentation and regular clinical examinations.

TREATMENT

The staging for melanoma is categorized by the tumor, node, metastasis (TNM) system.[13] Recommended treatment is wide local excision (1–2 cm) with margins dependent on Breslow depth. Breslow depth and risk factors such as mitotic rate and ulceration determine whether sentinel lymph node dissection is considered. Because controversy exists about when to offer sentinel lymph node dissection and recommendations are apt to change, clinicians are advised to access up-to-date guidelines on The National Comprehensive Cancer Network Web site (www.nccn.org)[14] (**Table 2**).

Table 2
Tumor, node, metastasis classification for cutaneous melanoma

Classification	Thickness (mm)	Ulceration/Mitoses
Tis	NA	NA
T1	≤1.00	a. Without ulceration and mitosis <1/mm² b. With ulceration or mitoses ≥1/mm²
T2	1.01–2.00	a. Without ulceration b. With ulceration
T3	2.01–4.00	a. Without ulceration b. With ulceration
T4	>4	a. Without ulceration b. With ulceration
N	Metastatic Nodes (N)	Nodal Metastatic Burden
N0	0	NA
N1	1	a. Micrometastasis b. Macrometastasis
N2	2–3	a. Micrometastasis b. Macrometastasis c. In transit metastases/satellites without metastatic nodes
N3	4+, or matted nodes, or in transit metastases/satellites with metastatic nodes	
M	Site	Serum LDH Level
M0	No distant metastases	NA
M1a	Distant skin, subcutaneous, or metastatic nodes	Normal
M1b	Lung metastases	Normal
M1c	All other visceral metastases Any distant metastases	Normal Increased

Abbreviations: LDH, lactate dehydrogenase; NA, not available.
From Amin MB, Edge SB, Greene FL, et al, editors. AJCC Cancer Staging Manual. 8th edition. New York: Springer: 2017; with permission.

NON MELANOMA SKIN MANCERS
Basal cell carcinoma

Genital basal cell carcinomas account for only 1% of cutaneous basal cell carcinomas. The average age at diagnosis is 73 years, with lesion size about 2 cm, arising most commonly on labia majora.[15] Pruritus is the most frequent symptom. Predisposing risk factors such as prior pelvic radiation therapy, chronic vulvar pruritus, and immunosuppression are present in about 20% of women with vulvar basal cell carcinoma. Vulvar basal cell carcinomas have a high recurrence rate (up to 20%) because of the large size and difficulty of complete excision.[16] Recommended treatment is simple excision without groin dissection because basal cell carcinomas rarely metastasize.[12]

PAGET DISEASE
Background

Paget disease accounts for 1% of vulvar malignancies and most commonly occurs in postmenopausal white women with an average age of 65 years. The mean size at diagnosis is approximately 4 cm, with a delay to diagnosis of 2 to 3 years. Like melanoma, vulvar Paget disease may be multifocal.[17] The lesion is typically a pruritic erythematous plaque with hyperkeratotic white scale. Only 10% of Paget disease is extramammary Paget disease (EMPD). About 80% of EMPD in women arises on the vulva. Invasion occurs in 16% to 19% of EMPD, with a clinically involved lymph node in about 15% of patients.[18] Paget disease is a neoplastic proliferation of oval cells with abundant pale cytoplasm, large nucleus, and prominent nucleoli. Paget cells stain with periodic acid–Schiff, carcinoembryonic antigen, and usually cytokeratin 7. Adnexal extension is frequent. A study showed follicular involvement in 93% of specimens, sebaceous gland involvement in 37%, and eccrine acrosyringeal involvement in 98% of cases.[19] Paget disease is divided into primary, secondary, microinvasive (≤1 mm), and invasive (>1 mm) (**Table 3**). Primary Paget disease is an intraepithelial adenocarcinoma with adnexal involvement with or without dermal invasion. Secondary Paget disease originates from an underlying noncutaneous adenocarcinoma and accounts for approximately 30% of genital Paget disease.[17] Multiple theories of the cause of Paget have been proposed, but none confirmed, so the cause remains unclear.

Diagnosis

Biopsy is essential for diagnosis. Any nonresolving erythematous hyperkeratotic or eroded plaque needs histologic sampling. If the entire plaque cannot be sampled because of size, multiple scouting biopsies are recommended in order to adequately assess for invasive disease. Fifteen percent of patients have a palpable lymph node at presentation requiring histologic assessment.[17] Complete evaluation for genital Paget disease includes a thorough history of genitourinary, gastrointestinal, and gynecologic symptoms to evaluate for an underlying carcinoma. A gynecologic examination is recommended plus additional examinations guided by pertinent symptoms. If the disease is localized to the vulva without an underlying carcinoma (EMPD), biopsy of involved skin to complete vulvar mapping is recommended. Photographic documentation of size and sites of involvement is helpful for clinical follow-up and evaluation. The pathology report should include depth of invasion in millimeters.[18]

Treatment

The most frequent treatment is wide local excision with consideration of inguinal femoral lymph node dissection if dermal invasion is greater than 1 mm. Neither sentinel lymph node excision nor inguinal femoral lymph node dissection is recommended for microinvasion (<1 mm). The subsequent morbidity of lymph node dissection, including lymphedema, leg pain, and impairment of sexual function, should be considered before sampling lymph nodes. Excision recurrence rates range from 21% to 61% even with uninvolved margins.[17]

Invasive Paget disease is treated with the same protocol as vulvar squamous cell carcinoma (SCC).[18] For noninvasive disease, imiquimod, a Toll-like receptor agonist, can be used to avoid the morbidity and decrease in sexual function associated with surgery. Studies report use from daily to 3 times a week for a duration of 5 to 26 weeks with almost 90% of patients having a response and 67% having a complete response.[18] A systematic review of the literature by Machida and colleagues[20] in 2015 found an overall 73% complete response rate and 17% persistent disease rate, and no disease progression on imiquimod. After imiquimod treatment, 6.5% of patients relapsed. Relapse did not correlate with age, primary versus recurrent disease, lesion size, frequency, or duration of imiquimod treatment. Common adverse

Table 3
Tumor, node, metastasis classification, carcinomas of vulva

T: Primary Tumor		
TX		Primary tumor cannot be assessed
T0		No primary tumor
Tis		Carcinoma in situ
T1	Tumor confined to vulva or vulva and perineum	
	T1a	Tumor 2 cm or less in greatest dimension and with stromal invasion $\leq$1.0 mm
	T1b	Tumor greater than 2 cm or with stromal invasion >1.0 mm
T2		Tumor of any size with extension to adjacent perineal structures: lower third urethra, lower third vagina, anus
T3 (T4 FIGO)		Tumor of any size with extension to the following structures: upper two-thirds urethra, upper two-thirds vagina, bladder mucosa, rectal mucosa, or fixed to pelvic bone
N: Regional Lymph Nodes		
NX	Regional	
NX		Regional nodes cannot be assessed
N0		No regional lymph node metastasis
N1		Lymph node metastasis with:
	N1a	1–2 lymph node metastases each <5 mm
	N1b	1 lymph node metastasis $\geq$5 mm
N2		Lymph node metastasis with:
	N2a	3 or more lymph node metastases each <5 mm
	N2b	2 or more lymph node metastases $\geq$5 mm
	N2c	Lymph node metastasis with extracapsular spread
N3		Fixed or ulcerated regional lymph node metastasis
M: Distant metastasis		
M0	None	
M1	Distant metastasis	

Abbreviation: FIGO, International Federation of Gynecology and Obstetrics.
From American Joint Committee on Cancer (AJCC). What is cancer staging? Available at: https://cancerstaging.org/references-tools/Pages/What-is-Cancer-Staging.aspx. Accessed April 21, 2017; with permission.

reactions, such as skin irritation, pain, and erosion, correlated with increased frequency of medication application. Imiquimod retains efficacy even in recurrent disease, with 75% of patients with recurrent Paget disease attaining complete response at 12 weeks after using imiquimod 3 times per week. Sixty-seven percent of patients relapsed in 5 to 72 months.[21] The depth of adnexal involvement in Paget disease may be responsible for recurrence rates because depth of involvement can reach 3.6 mm in the eccrine coils. Adnexal involvement is present in 90% of cases. The depth of penetration of imiquimod in the skin is unknown.[19] Laser is used to treat Paget disease with a high recurrence rate of 67% and with many of the morbidities of surgery. Topical steroids have no efficacy, and therefore no role in the treatment of Paget disease. Radiation therapy can be used as a primary treatment if surgery and imiquimod are not clinical options. Photodynamic therapy is used with a photosensitizer and red light but produces excessive pain without greater response than other options. Chemotherapy is indicated for metastatic disease.[17]

Prognosis

The overall survival is 100% for intraepithelial Paget disease and Paget disease with invasion less than 1 mm. For invasive disease greater than 1 mm, the overall survival rate is 15%. No data exist on the recurrence rate of vulvar Paget disease based on location or further stratification of depth of invasion. Risk of progression to invasive Paget disease is 3% after treatment, with a 2% risk of metastatic disease. Aggressive treatment should be avoided because the risk of recurrence is high, independent of treatment type, and risk of invasion and distant dissemination is low.[18]

Premalignant Vulvar Disease, High-Grade Intraepithelial Lesion, and Differential Vulvar Intraepithelial Neoplasia

The terminology of precancerous vulvar lesions has changed significantly in recent decades and is often a source of confusion for clinicians. In 1986 the International Society for the Study of Vulvovaginal Disease (ISSVD) introduced 2 types of squamous vulvar intraepithelial neoplasia (VIN): human papilloma virus (HPV)–associated VIN, graded 1 to 3; and differentiated VIN 3 (dVIN), which is non–HPV associated. In 2004, the ISSVD abandoned grading VIN as 1, 2, and 3, instead recommending VIN usual type (uVIN), which is HPV related, and VIN, differentiated type (dVIN), which is non–HPV related. VIN 1 was viewed as reactive change caused by HPV infection. In 2012, the American Society for Colposcopy and Cervical Pathology and the College of American Pathologists sponsored the Lower Anogenital Squamous Terminology (LAST) project to unify HPV squamous dysplasia terminology across the entire lower anogenital tract. LAST did not address non–HPV-related squamous dysplasia. LAST recommended the terms low-grade squamous intraepithelial lesion (LSIL) for flat condyloma or condyloma effect, not requiring therapy, and high-grade squamous intraepithelial lesion (HSIL) to refer to squamous dysplasia of the vulva, combining VIN 2 and 3 to create high-grade dysplasia that is easily reproducible. In 2014, the World Health Organization (WHO) published the fourth edition of *WHO Classification of Tumours of the Female Reproductive Organs*, which uses both LSIL, HSIL, and dVIN.[22] This discussion uses the terminology of the ISSVD 2015/WHO 2014 to refer to vulvar squamous dysplasia (**Table 4**).

Table 4
Different classifications of premalignant squamous lesions

WHO Classification 2014	1. LSIL 2. HSIL 3. dVIN
ISSVD Terminology 2015	1. LSIL = flat condyloma or HPV effect 2. HSIL = VIN usual type 3. dVIN
LAST 2012	1. LSIL: VIN1 2. HSIL: VIN2/VIN3

From Bornstein J, Bogliatto F, Haefner HK, et al. The 2015 International Society for the Study of Vulvovaginal Disease (ISSVD) terminology of vulvar squamous intraepithelial lesions. J Low Genit Tract Dis 2016;20(1):12; with permission.

HIGH-GRADE SQUAMOUS INTRAEPITHELIAL LESIONS

HSIL, referred to as uVIN or VIN2/VIN3 in the medical literature, is the most commonly diagnosed type of vulvar squamous dysplasia and has increased in incidence over the last 2 decades, although the incidence of invasive vulvar SCC has not increased.[23]

Greater than 80% of HSIL is HPV related, usually HPV16, whereas 90% of LSIL, condyloma effect, is caused by HPV 6 and 11.[23] Ninety-two percent of HSIL is caused by a single HPV type rather than multiple infections.[3] LSIL is treated as condyloma and does not represent true squamous dysplasia but is condyloma effect or reactive atypia. HSIL occurs most commonly in young women who smoke or have a history of multiple sexual partners, and is often multifocal. On histology, HSIL presents with crowded basophilic cells with mitotic figures, apoptotic cells, and dysmaturation involving greater than one-third of the epithelial thickness with blocklike p16 staining (a surrogate for HPV infection). From 3% to 5% of HSIL is thought to progress to invasive SCC if treated. Untreated, the risk of progression is closer to 10%.[24] Almost all invasive SCC is of the warty or basaloid subtypes and less often the keratinizing subtype.

Immunosuppression and advanced age favor progression of HSIL. HSIL presents as white to erythematous macules to papules on the introitus and labia minora. There is a high rate of HSIL and concurrent cervical dysplasia. HSIL can spontaneously regress (about 1%), most often reported in young pregnant women.

HIGH-GRADE SQUAMOUS INTRAEPITHELIAL LESION TREATMENT

Because HSIL maybe multicentric, documentation of disease, optimally with photography and biopsy mapping to evaluate extent of disease and evaluate for occult invasion, is recommended. Multiple treatment modalities exist, but simple excision with 5-mm margins is most common. Because HSIL extends down adnexae in hair-bearing skin, excision needs to include a depth of 4 mm. In non–hair-bearing skin, a depth of 1 mm is sufficient. The importance of margin distance is unclear, because one report found a recurrence rate of 46% in 22 months with positive margins, but a recurrence rate of 27% in 44 months even with negative margins.[3] Progression of disease is not influenced by radical excision of HSIL.[25] CO_2 laser is a second option but lacks the assessment of occult invasion, and the recurrence rate is equivalent to excision. Destruction from CO_2 laser needs to reach a depth of 4 mm to treat adnexal extension. Unexpected invasion is reported to occur in 3% to 19% of HSIL/dVIN biopsies.[23] Imiquimod 5% is a nondestructive option, without the risk of scarring which can result in psychosexual dysfunction.

Imiquimod is equally effective in all HPV subtype infections, working through Toll-like receptors to shift the immune response to type 1 T cell–mediated immunity. Histologic regression is strongly correlated with viral clearance.[25] Imiquimod is applied 2 to 4 times per week. One study found an 81% response rate with 35% complete response at 16 weeks. Complete responders remained disease free at 1 year. Close monitoring is required because progression, although rare, can occur even during treatment.[25] Terlou and colleagues[26] found that 88% of their complete responders were disease free at 7 years, with lesion size inversely correlated with complete response. Frequency of imiquimod application is limited by the adverse effects of erosion, skin irritation, and pain. Most patients tolerate application without needing dose reduction at a frequency of 3 to 4 times a week for 12 to 20 weeks. Nonresponsive lesions require excision to evaluate for invasion. Close clinical follow-up of treated areas is essential to evaluate for recurrence. The clear benefit of imiquimod treatment is avoiding alteration of vulvar architecture and the resultant psychosexual dysfunction. However, the depth of penetration of imiquimod in the skin is unknown, so it is uncertain whether adnexal extension of HSIL can be adequately treated with imiquimod.[19] For HSIL in human immunodeficiency virus, cidofovir has a reported efficacy of 51% but is still under study.[27] Clinical follow-up, regardless of treatment type, every 3 months for 2 to 3 years and then every 6 months is recommended.[3]

DIFFERENTIATED VULVAR INTRAEPITHELIAL NEOPLASIA

Although only accounting for 5% of vulvar dysplasia diagnoses, dVIN has a higher rate of progression to SCC, shorter time interval to progression, and higher recurrence rate than HSIL (**Table 5**). dVIN is diagnosed adjacent to invasive non–HPV-related SCC in about 46% of SCC excisions. Despite being underdiagnosed, dVIN is recognized in 38% of women who subsequently develop vulvar SCC. Seventy-five percent of the invasive cancers in these women developed in the same region as dVIN. Almost all SCC arising from dVIN is keratinizing.[29] dVIN is underdiagnosed, so dVIN should always be considered and biopsied in any nonresolving papule or plaque in chronic dermatoses such as LS and lichen planus.

Diagnosis

dVIN typically presents as a treatment-resistant hyperkeratotic plaque within the background of an inflammatory dermatosis, most frequently LS. Instead of presenting

Table 5
Comparison between differentiated vulvar intraepithelial neoplasia and high-grade intraepithelial lesion

	dVIN	HSIL
Age	Sixth–eighth decade	Third–fifth decade
Percentage of all Vulvar Precancer Diagnoses	5	95
Multifocality	Unusual	>50%
Smoking	Not associated	60% smokers
Associated Conditions	Chronic inflammatory dermatoses, most commonly lichen sclerosis Only 1.5% dVIN is HPV+	>80% HPV+ HPV 16%–77% of HSIL HPV 33%–10% HPV18%–2.5%
Pigmented Clinically	Unknown	10%
Percentage that Progress to Carcinoma	35%	5%
Time from Biopsy to Invasion (mo)	23	41
Recurrence	Common	Less common than dVIN, but significant at 15%–50%
Immunohistochemistry	Commonly p53+ basal and suprabasal layers	p16 block positivity
Adnexal Extension (Into Follicles, Sebaceous Glands)	Rare	Common
Most Common Invasion Histology if Progresses	Keratinizing SCC	Warty/basaloid SCC

Data from Refs.[3,23,24,28]

as a hyperkeratotic plaque, dVIN can be indistinguishable from the background dermatosis. Alternate clinical morphologies of dVIN include spongiotic and atrophic papules further complicating clinical diagnosis. Women with vulvar LS and lichen planus are at higher risk for dVIN and SCC and require close follow-up monitoring.[30] Lifelong monitoring is recommended for all patients with LS because risk of SCC increases with duration of LS: 1% at 2 years and 37% after 25 years of disease.[31] Other studies found that the rate of progression of LS ranged from 2% to 5% but duration of disease was not studied.[32] Lee and colleagues[33] found that the only risk factor for progression from LS to vulvar SCC was noncompliance with LS treatment. Photographic documentation of vulvar LS, lichen planus, and other chronic vulvar dermatoses, to monitor treatment-resistant areas, should be considered.

Biopsies may not adequately sample dVIN, leading to delayed diagnosis because the histologic features of dVIN are often subtle and histologic diagnosis is aided by including normal adjacent skin for comparison. Van den Eiden and colleagues[34] found atypical basal mitotic figures, basal atypia, dyskeratosis, prominent nucleoli and elongation and anastomosis of the rete as histologic features diagnostic of dVIN, with basal atypia being most predictive. P53 staining may be helpful because 83% of dVIN stains with p53, in the basal and suprabasal layers. However, a subset of dVIN is p53 negative. Rare cases of dVIN present as full-thickness keratinocyte atypia, similar to HSIL, but HPV negative, further complicating the histologic diagnosis of dVIN.[23] In addition, histologic concordance of the diagnosis of dVIN is low, leading to delayed or missed diagnosis.[34] Excision is the treatment of choice because of the necessity of evaluating for occult invasion.[24] Clinical follow-up every 3 months for 2 to 3 years and then every 6 months is recommended.[3]

SQUAMOUS CELL CARCINOMA

Although the prevalences of dVIN and HSIL have increased in the past 2 decades, the incidence of vulvar SCC remains stable at 1 to 2 per 100,000 women.[32] The diagnosis of SCC is often delayed, even in symptomatic women. A study by Rhodes and colleagues[35] found a delay of more than 1 year in 22% of women. Two causal pathways to vulvar carcinoma exist: an HPV-related and a non–HPV-related pathway. HPV-related SCC arises in younger women (63 years) and accounts for 20% of invasive disease versus non–HPV-related SCC (70 years), which accounts for 80% of invasive disease.[3,32] Inguinofemoral node status is the most important prognostic factor in vulvar SCC.[36] Invasive SCC is staged according to TNM and International Federation of Gynecology and Obstetrics (FIGO) staging systems. Stage 1a disease has less than a 1% risk of metastasis[23] (see **Table 3**).

Treatment

First-line treatment is excision with or without sentinel lymph node dissection. Lymph node dissection is omitted for patients with clinically negative nodes, unilateral disease, tumor size less than 2 cm, and stromal invasion less than 1 mm. Excision margins of 8 to 10 mm are sufficient, with no increased survival for margins greater than 10 mm.[37] For patients with tumors less than 4 cm, unilateral, and more than 2 cm from the midline, sentinel lymph node dissection is an option. Midline tumors need bilateral sentinel lymph node dissection and, if sentinel nodes are not identified, then bilateral inguinofemoral lymph node dissection is required. If sentinel nodes are positive, inguinofemoral node dissection is performed. The false-negative sentinel lymph node dissection rate is 2% to 6% for tumors less than 4 cm. The risk for groin recurrence is greatest in tumors larger than 2 cm and midline tumors. Mortality is high for groin recurrences.[38] The number of involved lymph nodes inversely correlates with prognosis, as does the presence of extracapsular growth. Lymph node involvement requires adjuvant radiation therapy.[37]

However, radiation offers no clear benefit to patients with 1 positive node if nodal tumor involvement is less than 5 mm.[39] If 3 or more unilateral inguinofemoral nodes contain tumor or if nodal macrometastases (>10 mm) or extracapsular extension is present, then pelvic node dissection is performed.[40] Tumor size is inversely correlated with prognosis, with tumors less than 6 cm having a 5-year overall survival of around 78%. The overall survival decreases precipitously to 36% in tumors greater than 6 cm.[37] In the past 2 decades, there has been no improvement in therapy for advanced vulvar SCC or recurrent disease. It is unclear whether chemotherapy or radiation and chemotherapy is most effective as an adjuvant treatment.[41] Reversible tyrosine kinase inhibitors are being studied for advanced/recurrent disease.[40] Clinicians are advised to access up-to-date guidelines on The National Comprehensive Cancer Network Web site (www.nccn.org).[14]

REFERENCES

1. Gleason BC, Hirsch MS, Nucci MR, et al. Atypical genital nevi. Am J Surg Pathol 2008;32(1):51–7.
2. Ribé A. Melanocytic lesions of the genital area with attention given to atypical genital nevi. J Cutan Pathol 2008;35:24–7.
3. Preti M, Scurry J, Marchitelli CE, et al. Vulvar intraepithelial neoplasia. Best Pract Res Clin Obstet Gynaecol 2014;28(7):1051–62.
4. Edwards L. Pigmented vulvar lesions. Dermatol Ther 2010;23(5):449–57.
5. Rouzbahman M, Kamel-Reid S, Al Habeeb A, et al. Malignant melanoma of vulva and vagina. J Low Genit Tract Dis 2015;19(4):350–3.
6. Lenane P, Keane CO, Connell BO, et al. Genital melanotic macules: clinical, histologic, immunohistochemical, and ultrastructural features. J Am Acad Dermatol 2000;42(4):640–4.
7. Murzaku EC, Penn LA, Hale CS, et al. Vulvar nevi, melanosis, and melanoma: an epidemiologic, clinical, and histopathologic review. J Am Acad Dermatol 2014; 71(6):1241–9.
8. Duffy K, Grossman D. The dysplastic nevus: from historical perspective to management in the modern era. J Am Acad Dermatol 2012;67(1):19.e1-12.
9. Carlson JA, Mu XC, Slominski A, et al. Melanocytic proliferations associated with lichen sclerosus. Arch Dermatol 2002;138(1):77–87.
10. Vyas R, Thompson CL, Zargar H, et al. Epidemiology of genitourinary melanoma in the United States: 1992 through 2012. J Am Acad Dermatol 2016;75(1): 144–50.
11. Iacoponi S, Rubio P, Garcia E, et al. Prognostic factors of recurrence and survival in vulvar melanoma. Int J Gynecol Cancer 2016;26(7):1307–12.
12. Pleunis N, Schuurman MS, Van Rossum MM, et al. Rare vulvar malignancies; incidence, treatment and survival in the Netherlands. Gynecol Oncol 2016;142(3): 440–5.
13. Balch CM, Gershenwald JE, Soong S, et al. Final version of 2009 AJCC melanoma staging and classification. J Clin Oncol 2009;27(36):6199–206.
14. Network NCC. Evidence-based cancer guidelines, oncology drug compendium, oncology continuing medical education. Available at: http://www.nccn.org. Accessed January 29, 2017.

15. Pisani C, Poggiali S, Padova L, et al. Basal cell carcinoma of the vulva. J Eur Acad Dermatol Venereol 2006;20(4):446–8.

16. Gibson GE, Ahmed I. Perianal and genital basal cell carcinoma: A clinicopathologic review of 51 cases. J Am Acad Dermatol 2001;45(1):68–71.

17. Iacoponi S, Zalewski K, Fruscio R, et al. Prognostic factors for recurrence and survival among patients with invasive vulvar Paget disease included in the VULCAN study. Int J Gynaecol Obstet 2016;133(1):76–9.

18. van der Linden M, Meeuwis KAP, Bulten J, et al. Paget disease of the vulva. Crit Rev Oncol Hematol 2016;101:60–74.

19. Konstantinova AM, Shelekhova KV, Stewart CJ, et al. Depth and patterns of adnexal involvement in primary extramammary (anogenital) Paget disease. Am J Dermatopathol 2016;38(11):802–8.

20. Machida H, Moeini A, Roman LD, et al. Effects of imiquimod on vulvar Paget's disease: a systematic review of literature. Gynecol Oncol 2015;139(1):165–71.

21. Cowan RA, Black DR, Hoang LN, et al. A pilot study of topical imiquimod therapy for the treatment of recurrent extramammary Paget's disease. Gynecol Oncol 2016;142(1):139–43.

22. Bornstein J, Bogliatto F, Haefner HK, et al. The 2015 ISSVD terminology of vulvar squamous intraepithelial lesions. J Low Genit Tract Dis 2016;20(2):190.

23. Hoang LN, Park KJ, Soslow RA, et al. Squamous precursor lesions of the vulva: current classification and diagnostic challenges. Pathology 2016;48(4):291–302.

24. van de Nieuwenhof HP, van der Avoort IAM, de Hullu JA. Review of squamous premalignant vulvar lesions. Crit Rev Oncol Hematol 2008;68(2):131–56.

25. van Seters M, van Beurden M, ten Kate FJW, et al. Treatment of vulvar intraepithelial neoplasia with topical imiquimod. N Engl J Med 2008;358(14):1465–73.

26. Terlou A, van Seters M, Ewing PC, et al. Treatment of vulvar intraepithelial neoplasia with topical imiquimod: Seven years median follow-up of a randomized clinical trial. Gynecol Oncol 2011;121(1):157–62.

27. Stier EA, Goldstone SE, Einstein MH, et al. Safety and efficacy of topical cidofovir to treat high-grade perianal and vulvar intraepithelial neoplasia in HIV-positive men and women. AIDS 2013;27(4):545–51.

28. Nugent EK, Brooks RA, Barr CD, et al. Clinical and pathologic features of vulvar intraepithelial neoplasia in premenopausal and postmenopausal women. J Low Genit Tract Dis 2011;15(1):15–9.

29. Bigby SM, Eva LJ, Fong KL, et al. The natural history of vulvar intraepithelial neoplasia, differentiated type. Int J Gynecol Pathol 2016;35(6):574–84.

30. Regauer S, Reich O, Eberz B. Vulvar cancers in women with vulvar lichen planus: a clinicopathological study. J Am Acad Dermatol 2014;71(4):698–707.

31. Micheletti L, Preti M, Radici G, et al. Vulvar lichen sclerosus and neoplastic transformation. J Low Genit Tract Dis 2016;20(2):180–3.

32. van de Nieuwenhof HP, Bulten J, Hollema H, et al. Differentiated vulvar intraepithelial neoplasia is often found in lesions, previously diagnosed as lichen sclerosus, which have progressed to vulvar squamous cell carcinoma. Mod Pathol 2010;24(2):297–305.

33. Lee A, Bradford J, Fischer G. Long-term management of adult vulvar lichen sclerosus. JAMA Dermatol 2015;151(10):1061.

34. van den Einden LC, de Hullu JA, Massuger LF, et al. Interobserver variability and the effect of education in the histopathological diagnosis of differentiated vulvar intraepithelial neoplasia. Mod Pathol 2013;26(6):874–80.

35. Rhodes CA, Cummins C, Shafi MI. The management of squamous cell vulval cancer: a population based retrospective study of 411 cases. Br J Obstet Gynaecol 1998;105(2):200–5.
36. Luchini C, Nottegar A, Solmi M, et al. Prognostic implications of extranodal extension in node-positive squamous cell carcinoma of the vulva: a systematic review and meta-analysis. Surg Oncol 2016;25(1):60–5.
37. Aragona AM, Cuneo NA, Soderini AH, et al. An analysis of reported independent prognostic factors for survival in squamous cell carcinoma of the vulva: is tumor size significance being underrated? Gynecol Oncol 2014;132(3):643–8.
38. Klapdor R, Hertel H, Soergel P, et al. Groin recurrences in node negative vulvar cancer patients after sole sentinel lymph node dissection. Int J Gynecol Cancer 2017;27(1):166–70.
39. Micheletti L, Preti M. Surgery of the vulva in vulvar cancer. Best Pract Res Clin Obstet Gynaecol 2014;28(7):1074–87.
40. Alkatout I, Günther V, Schubert M, et al. Vulvar cancer: epidemiology, clinical presentation, and management options. Int J Womens Health 2015;7:305–13.
41. Reade CJ, Eiriksson LR, Mackay H. Systemic therapy in squamous cell carcinoma of the vulva: current status and future directions. Gynecol Oncol 2014;132(3):780–9.

Red Rashes of the Vulva

Lynne H. Morrison, MD[a],*, Catherine M. Leclair, MD[b]

KEYWORDS

- Vulvar dermatitis • Vulvar infections • Vulvar neoplasm • Vulvar skin disease

KEY POINTS

- Vulvar skin disease may present as red rash. The unique nature of mixed skin makes it difficult to secure a diagnosis because classic disease features may be absent.
- Neoplasms of the vulva include Paget's disease, low-grade squamous intraepithelial lesion/high-grade squamous intraepithelial lesion associated with human papilloma virus infection, and differentiated vulvar intraepithelial neoplasia often associated with lichen sclerosus.
- Inflammatory skin diseases of the vulva can present as a red rash, including the diagnoses of psoriasis, seborrheic dermatitis, contact dermatitis, and eczema.
- Infectious red patches or plaques often associated with itch and burn are tinea, candidiasis, perianal streptococcus, and erythrasma.

Red patches and plaques of the vulva may be manifestations of neoplasms, infections or inflammatory skin diseases including contact dermatitis, psoriasis, seborrheic dermatitis, differentiated vulvar intraepithelial neoplasia (dVIN), low- or high-grade squamous intra-epithelial lesion (LSIL/HSIL), Paget disease, candidal, fungal or bacterial infections. These diseases can mimic one another clinically and features that generally allow the diseases to be identified on most cutaneous surfaces can be altered in the moist, occluded vulvar environment, making clinical diagnosis difficult. A detailed history and thorough physical examination can point to the likely diagnosis, but biopsy and culture may be needed for diagnosis especially in refractory disease. It is not uncommon for several of these processes to be present concomitantly or complicating other vulvar diseases.

NEOPLASMS

Squamous Intraepithelial Lesions of the Vulva: High and Low-grade Squamous Intraepithelial Lesions of the Vulva and Differentiated Vulvar Intraepithelial Neoplasms

Squamous intraepithelial lesions of the vulva and squamous cell carcinoma (SCC) of the vulva represent neoplastic change of the epithelium and are derived from one of

Disclosure statement: The authors have nothing to disclose.
[a] Department of Dermatology, Oregon Health & Science University, 3303 Southwest Bond Avenue, CH16D, Portland, OR 97239, USA; [b] Program in Vulvar Health, Division of General Obstetrics & Gynecology, Oregon Health & Science University, 3181 Southwest Sam Jackson Park Road, UHN 50, Portland, OR 97239, USA
* Corresponding author.
E-mail address: MORRISOL@OHSU.EDU

Obstet Gynecol Clin N Am 44 (2017) 353–370
http://dx.doi.org/10.1016/j.ogc.2017.05.002
0889-8545/17/© 2017 Elsevier Inc. All rights reserved.

obgyn.theclinics.com

2 pathways. These lesions stem either from human papilloma virus (HPV) disease or from inflammatory skin diseases (ie, lichen sclerosus) of the vulva. For some time, terminology of vulvar lesions has not differentiated between these two pathways nor has it distinguished those lesions with greater malignant potential. Lesions were classified as VIN1, 2, or 3 with the assumption that there was a graduation of disease from 1 to 3. This classification led to the overdiagnosis and overtreatment of low-grade disease (ie, VIN1) and a misunderstanding of the HPV effect on the vulva.

In 2012, the original Lower Anogenital Squamous Terminology (LAST) criteria were published in hopes of creating a consensus terminology for the effects of HPV disease of the vulva[1] (**Table 1**). This consensus process was created to recommend terminology reflecting histopathologic changes that were acceptable to all specialties managing disease of the lower genital tract. However, in 2015 this terminology was modified to reflect the differences in malignant potential between the two disease pathways.[2] Eighty percent of squamous cancers of the vulva are not HPV derived but originate from coexisting inflammatory skin disease, such as lichen sclerosus (LS) with dVIN as the precursor lesion.[2,3] The risk of SCC in women with LS is approximately 5%,[4,5] double to triple that of the unaffected population. The remaining 20% are derived from HPV diseases of the vulva and represent a progression from HSIL of the vulva. Although dVIN was accepted by the International Society for the Study of Vulvovaginal Disease's (ISSVD) Vulvar Oncology Committee in 2004[3] as a lesion of malignant potential, it was not recognized by the original LAST criteria. The absence led to modification of terminology by the World Health Organization and the ISSVD to include dVIN as a lesion with malignant potential distinct from HSIL of the vulva and republication of the LAST in 2015.[2] In addition, emphasis was placed on differentiating HPV-derived low- and high-grade lesions as different lesions, as a matter of underscoring that low-grade lesions had little malignant potential and may never progress to a high-grade lesion. The updated LAST criteria now reflect the most updated terminology of lesions of the vulva.[2]

HPV is a large family of DNA viruses that can infect the lower genital tract and is associated with benign, precancerous, and malignant neoplasms of the cervix, vulva, vagina, and anus. Risk is divided into low- and high-risk HPV subtypes (**Table 2**), with high-risk subtypes having the greatest potential for malignancy. Low-risk subtypes are most commonly associated with anogenital warts or flat condyloma (condyloma acuminata) or lesions with an HPV effect. This lesion is no longer referenced as VIN1 but as LSIL of the vulva (low-grade intraepithelial lesion). It is understood to have low malignant potential and does not necessarily need treatment.[2,5,6] High-grade subtypes are most commonly associated with palpable and/or visible lesions of the vulva. These lesions are associated with 20% of SCC of the vulva and need treatment.[4–6] HSIL often occurs in younger woman than dVIN, with classic demographics of smoking, multiple sex partners, and early age of sexual activity.

Table 1			
Comparison of terminology for vulvar intraepithelial lesions			
Year	**1980**	**2012**	**2015**
Terminology	VIN1	LSIL (VIN1)	LSIL/condyloma
	VIN2	HSIL (VIN2/3)	HSIL
	VIN3		dVIN

Table 2 Human papilloma virus low-risk and high-risk viral subtypes	
Low-Risk Subtypes	**High-Risk Subtypes**
6, 11, 40, 42, 43, 44, 53, 54, 61, 72, 73, and 81	16, 18, 31, 33, 35, 39, 45, 51, 2, 56, 59, and 68

Women with condyloma/LSIL/HSIL/dVIN can present with a host of symptoms. About 40% of women will be symptom free. Pruritus, burning, pain, and irritation are common symptoms. Bulky warts can interfere with defecation and sexual intercourse.

Physical examination can be challenging to visibly differentiate low- and high-grade lesions. Thus, the only true way to distinguish is to gain histologic confirmation with biopsy. Condyloma has a typical verrucous appearance with an exophytic papule (**Fig. 1**). LSIL/flat condyloma may be a smooth, confluent patch or plaque that may be erythematous or white. If the lesion is pruritic, there may be accompanying signs of excoriation. High-grade lesions may be gray, white, or erythematous. Associated fissures, erosions, or ulcerations are more concerning signs and biopsy should be considered. HSIL may present as a single lesion or be multifocal. Firmness may represent extension beyond the epithelium; therefore, a biopsy should be obtained (**Figs. 2** and **3**).

dVIN exists in a background of inflammatory skin disease, with the most common being LS. It is not uncommon for women who present with vulvar SCC to have LS that has been undiagnosed and/or untreated. Lesions that are firm, eroded, ulcerated, and resistant to treatment (for LS) should be considered for biopsy to rule out SCC because it is difficult to distinguish dVIN from SCC (**Figs. 4** and **5**). (See Vyas' article, "Genital Lichen Sclerosus and its Mimics," in this issue, for details regarding diagnosis and treatment of that inflammatory skin disease.)

Treatment of low-grade squamous intraepithelial lesion/condyloma
Most LSIL do not need to be treated and will resolve spontaneously over months.[6–9] The misunderstanding that LSIL (previously VIN1) is a progressive condition has led to overtreatment with physical and emotional ramifications. Close follow-up with physical examination is ideal for patients with LSIL and is considered the primary treatment.

In contrast, most women with condyloma will often opt for treatment. Although 20% to 30% of warts will regress, most will persist or progress. Treatment goals are to

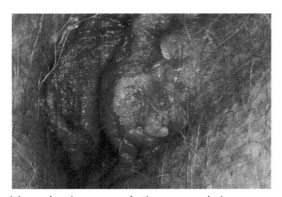

Fig. 1. Vulvar condyloma showing an exophytic verrucous lesion.

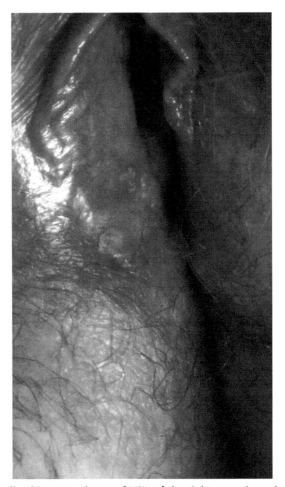

Fig. 2. Single, small, white-gray plaque of HSIL of the right posterior vulva.

eradicate the lesions while maintaining normal anatomy and function of the individual. There are both clinician-administered and patient-administered treatment choices. Options include cyto-destructive techniques, immune therapy, and surgical eradication. Treatment selection is based on a frank discussion between patients and practitioner with consideration of patient compliance, provider experience, side effect profile, cost, patient convenience, anatomic site, and the size/number/morphology of the lesions. Most treatment options are equally efficacious and require multiple applications. None confers benefit over another. Bulky warts may need a combination of more than one strategy, such as surgical excision and topical immune therapy (**Table 3**).[7–9]

Treatment of high-grade squamous intraepithelial lesion/differentiated vulvar intraepithelial neoplasia

HSIL/dVIN are high-grade lesions that require treatment. Ones that are raised, ulcerated, and have irregular borders are suspicious for SCC and should be excised rather than ablated or chemically treated. Additionally, if a woman has risks for

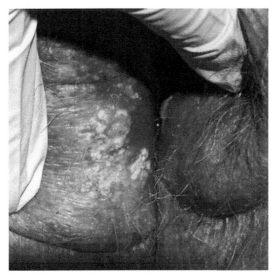

Fig. 3. HSIL and invasive SCC with erosion.

SCC, such as previous cancer, smoker, LS, or immunosuppression, consideration should be given to excision first because this provides both diagnostic and therapeutic benefit. The mainstay of treatment of HSIL/dVIN is surgical with options, including wide local excision and skinning vulvectomy. Laser ablation is also an option but

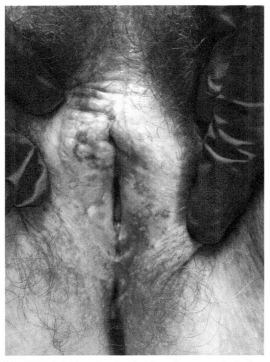

Fig. 4. Severe LS with dVIN right hemi-vulva (white plaque posterior).

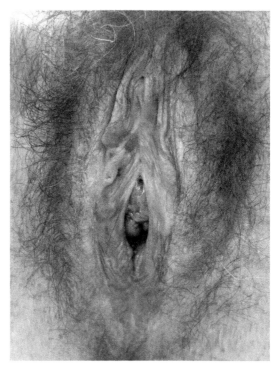

Fig. 5. Severe LS with dVIN upper right labia minora with erosion.

does not provide a tissue sample for histologic review. Data support the use of immunotherapy with topical imiquimod (Aldara) to be as effective as surgery. Imiquimod is ideal in a young woman with multifocal HSIL disease who would like to avoid a potentially disfiguring procedure, such as a skinning vulvectomy.[4,6,9,10]

Paget Disease of the Vulva

Extramammary Paget disease (EMPD) is a rare intraepidermal adenocarcinoma, most common in Caucasian women in their 60s and 70s. EMPD most often involves the vulva but can also affect the perineal skin, perianal skin, and axillae. EMPD has been reported to be associated with underlying dermal adnexal neoplasms and with coexisting internal malignancies often of the breast and the gastrointestinal and genitourinary tract.[11,12]

Table 3
Treatment options for condyloma

Cyto-Destructive	Immune Therapy	Surgical
Podophyllin and podofilox[a]	Imiquimod[a]	Excision
Trichloroacetic acid	5-Fluorouracil	Electrodesiccation
Cryotherapy		Laser
Sinecatechins[a]		

[a] Patient applied.

EMPD may be classified into either in primary cutaneous or secondary non-cutaneous forms. In primary EMPD, the malignant cells may arise from intraepidermal portions of apocrine or eccrine glands, stem cells, or mammarylike glands resulting in an intraepidermal neoplasm. Primary EMPD may become invasive and metastasize to local lymph nodes and distant sites. Secondary EMPD is thought to arise from epidermotropic spread of cells from underlying dermal adnexal gland adenocarcinomas or, in approximately 15% to 30% of cases, malignancies of the gastrointestinal or urogenital tract.[13] EMPD often extends beyond clinically apparent margins, which makes removal of disease without overtreatment challenging. Various interventions are described, including Mohs micrographic surgery, radiation therapy, photo dynamic therapy, topical imiquimod (immunotherapy), and laser therapy, with little agreement regarding the specific role of each treatment. Recurrence is common, necessitating long-term surveillance.

Typical symptoms include irritation, itching, and burning, although approximately 5% to 15% of patients are asymptomatic at the time of diagnosis. Often, vulvar Paget disease is not suspected early in the course of disease; multiple therapies are tried before a biopsy is done to establish a diagnosis, which can be delayed on average of 2 years. Because of the risk of associated internal malignancies, a thorough history and review of systems, including vulvovaginal, gastrointestinal, and urologic symptoms, should be obtained early.[11–13]

The most commonly affected site is the vulva, followed by perineal and perianal skin, and, less commonly, the axilla, buttocks, thighs, and eyelids. The primary lesion of vulvar EMPD may be solitary or multiple, well-demarcated scaling plaques, which may be pink or red, with areas of hypopigmentation or hyperpigmentation, which has been referred to as having a strawberries and cream appearance. Some demonstrate erosions, crusting, and ulceration. Nodules, papillomatous change, or lymphadenopathy may also be present (**Fig. 6**).

In view of potential associations with underlying malignancy, a complete physical examination should include:[13,14]

- Complete skin examination
- Complete general physical examination
- Palpation of lymph nodes, liver, and spleen and clinical breast examination
- Digital rectal examination
- Gynecologic examination, including Papanicolaou test

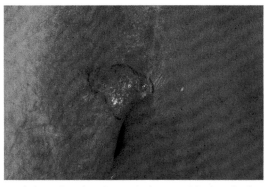

Fig. 6. Paget disease of the vulva showing red plaque with sharply demarcated edges and erosions.

The diagnosis of EMPD is established by skin biopsy. Histopathologic findings include intraepithelial collections of Paget cells (large round cells with abundant basophilic cytoplasm). Biopsies obtained for immunohistochemical staining may help differentiate primary from secondary forms of EMPD (in particular, markers CK 7 and CK 20), determine the location of underlying adenocarcinoma, and differentiate this from other conditions in the histopathologic differential diagnoses, such as Bowen disease, Langerhans cell histiocytosis, sebaceous carcinoma, Merkel cell carcinoma, and malignant melanoma.[14,15] Multiple additional biopsies of the affected skin (referred to as vulvar mapping) may help distinguish between invasive and noninvasive disease.

Reports in the literature vary widely regarding the incidence of underlying malignancies and which investigations are needed. Eleven percent to 54% of patients with vulvar Paget disease have been reported to have an associated underlying malignancy.[14] In general, guidelines, including those of the American College of Obstetrics and Gynecology and Royal College of Obstetricians and Gynecologists, advise evaluation of breasts and the genitourinary and gastrointestinal tract.[14] This evaluation may be best done by a gynecologic oncologist.

Treatment can be pharmacologic, nonpharmacologic, and surgical. Pharmacologic treatments include:[8,13,14]

- Imiquimod which is an immune response modulator that stimulates cytokine production where applied. The reported treatment frequency is most often 3 to 4 times weekly, with duration ranging from 4 to 26 weeks. Benefit in noninvasive vulvar Paget disease may be as high as 88% clinical response. Side effects include local inflammation and pain.[14]
- Topical 5-fluorouracil (5-FU) which is used with a variety of regimens. As a sole therapy, it can induce clinical clearing but not histopathologic eradication of disease. It is mostly used in combination with surgery.
- Topical 3.5% bleomycin ointment, applied twice daily for 2 weeks, followed by a 4- to 6-week rest period for a total of 4 cycles, has shown a benefit in a small number of patients with recurrent vulvar EMPD.

Nonpharmacologic therapies include:[11,13,14]

- Photodynamic therapy (PDT), a physical modality using a photosensitizing agent applied to the skin followed by irradiation with visible red light to activate the agent, generating reactive oxygen species. PDT has been used alone and in combination with surgery, laser, and radiation. Although topical agents may not reach deep appendageal disease, intravenous porphyrin circumvents this. Efficacy is not well documented because of disease and treatment variation. Case series with short-term follow-up report complete and partial response for vulvar EMPD.
- Radiation therapy has been used as primary treatment of invasive and noninvasive vulvar EMPD and for recurrent disease after surgery and adjuvant to surgery. Long-term follow-up shows recurrence rates less than 20% with remissions lasting as long as 6 to 8 years.[16]
- Carbon dioxide and Nd:YAG laser therapy has been used for recurrence after surgery or in combination with PDT. Limitations include lack of clear surgical margins or identification of invasive disease and the possibility that superficial ablation may miss disease extending to adnexal and follicular structures. Although complete response is possible, significant recurrences can occur.

Surgery is considered standard treatment of vulvar EMPD.[11,13,14]

- Surgery consists mostly of wide local excision, with the goal of obtaining clear margins. However, because of multicentricity and invasion into skin that appears clinically normal, accurate determination of surgical margins can be difficult.
- All procedures, including radical resections, suffer from high local recurrence rates, which can be well more than 30% for invasive as well as noninvasive disease and as high as 44%.
- Mohs micrographic surgery (MMS) can reduce local recurrence rates and preserve tissue. In 2 studies, recurrence rates after MMS were 8% to 23% versus 22% to 33% following conventional surgery.[17]
- Some investigators recommend inguinofemoral lymphadenectomy when invasive vulvar Paget disease is greater than 1 mm in depth. The less invasive sentinel lymph node biopsy has been suggested for all EMPD, except those with strictly intraepidermal disease.[13]
- Surgical complications include infection, hematoma, and wound dehiscence as well as potential long-term sexual dysfunction and decreased quality of life.
- Lymphadenectomy presents additional complications, such as lymphocyst formation and development of lymphedema, cellulitis, and leg pain.

PDT, radiation, 5-FU, bleomycin, and laser are often used as combination therapy, either together or especially after surgery.

The prognosis for primary EMPD localized to the epithelium is excellent, with a 5-year survival of 95% to 100%. However, disease with deeper than 1-mm invasion carries a much lower survival rate. Van der Linden,[14] summarizing 11 series, found the following death rates:

- 2 of 246 (4.9%) with noninvasive EMPD
- 0 of 19 (0%) with invasion less than or equal to 1 mm
- 16 of 55 (29.1%) with invasion greater than 1 mm

The prognosis of secondary EMPD depends on that of the underlying malignancy but overall is worse than for primary disease.

There are no guidelines for the frequency of follow-up or subsequent internal malignancy screening in EMPD. However, because recurrences have been detected as long as 15 years after initial diagnosis, long-term surveillance for both local recurrence and associated malignancies is necessary, with a low threshold for biopsying any suspicious lesions.

INFLAMMATORY
Psoriasis

Psoriasis is an inflammatory skin condition that can affect the vulva. The condition affects approximately 1% to 2% of the population with an unclear cause. In the vulva, psoriasis usually does not have classic silvery patches and plaques like those seen on extensor surfaces and the scalp but manifests as bright erythematous, sharply demarcated patches, and plaques that may be confluent. Silvery plaques may be seen on the mons but are not usually present on the rest of the vulva (**Figs. 7** and **8**).

Women with vulvar psoriasis often present with pruritus. Women may report other conditions associated with psoriasis, such as inflammatory bowel disease, arthritis and dystrophy of the nails. Differential diagnosis for women presenting with these signs and symptoms include contact dermatitis, vulvovaginal candidiasis, eczema,

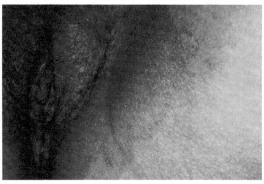

Fig. 7. Well-defined, red, scaling, thin plaque of psoriasis.

seborrheic dermatitis, cellulitis and tinea. Diagnosis is based on clinical presentation and biopsy. Examining the body for other signs of psoriatic plaques may help secure the diagnosis.

Topical corticosteroids are often the first-line treatment of vulvar psoriasis. Choice of potency of steroid is based on extent of symptoms and disease. Twice-daily or daily treatment with an ultrapotent steroid (group 1), such as clobetasol propionate 0.05% ointment, is recommended for 2 to 4 weeks in women with severe disease. Midpotency (group 4) or low potency (group 1) corticosteroids may be appropriate for mild-moderate disease or small areas of affected vulva (**Table 4**). Pulse with frequent twice daily or daily use and then tapering to twice weekly use is a strategy for treatment as opposed to as-needed use of medication. Close follow-up to monitor clinical response is appropriate, especially when a pulse of ultrahigh-potency topical steroid has been initiated. Decision to taper and discontinue versus maintenance treatment of the steroid is based on the desired goals of patients and clinical recommendation of the practitioner.

Other treatments for vulvar psoriasis, such as topical tacrolimus or pimecrolimus, vitamin D analogues, and systemic antiinflammatory medications, should be done in consultation with a dermatologist.

Seborrheic Dermatitis

Seborrheic dermatitis is a chronic inflammatory condition affecting areas of the body rich in sebaceous glands, such as the axilla, scalp, face, and upper trunk. Less commonly, it can also affect the vulva.

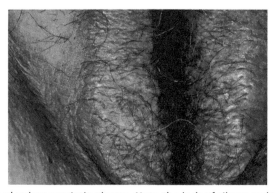

Fig. 8. Well-defined vulvar psoriatic plaque. Note the lack of silvery scale.

Table 4
Steroid grouping based on potency

Potency		
Ultrahigh (group 1)	Clobetasol 0.05% ointment	Halobetasol 0.05% ointment
High (group 2)	Betamethasone Dipropionate Ointment 0.05%	
Mid (group 4)	Flurandrenolide 0.05% ointment	Triamcinolone acetonide 0.1% ointment
Low (group 7)	Hydrocortisone 2.5% ointment	

Women classically present with an erythematous pruritic rash of the groin-vulva that is scaly and greasy appearing. It may present in other areas of the body, particularly the face and scalp (margins of the scalp, nasolabial folds, eyebrows, and outer ear), giving clues to the presence of seborrhea. Clinical suspicion, examination of other areas of the body, and occasionally biopsy are necessary to diagnose this disorder.

Seborrheic dermatitis is chronic and recurring. It exacerbates in times of stress. On the scalp, it is primarily controlled with dandruff shampoos that are selenium based (Selsen or Selsen Blue) or tar based (T-gel). In more sensitive skin of the groin-vulva, a mid to low potency topical corticosteroid is typically used (see **Table 4**).

Eczema

Eczema and dermatitis are interchangeable terms describing a morphologic group of skin diseases that share a common clinical appearance and histopathologic features but not a common cause.[18] The types of dermatitis relevant to vulvar area include allergic and irritant contact dermatitis (CD) and atopic and seborrheic dermatitis. Patients with atopic dermatitis are sometimes referred to as having eczema and are predisposed to irritant dermatitis and skin infections due to impaired barrier function inherent to atopic skin.[19]

All types of dermatitis present with variable itching, burning, or rawness. Clinically, dermatitis appears as red, scaling plaques with ill-defined borders and epidermal disruption (minute erosions resulting from rupture of subclinical epidermal vesicles) on the surface. Scaling may be less apparent in the vulvar area because of the occluded, moist nature of skin in this location. Irritant and allergic CD occur at the site of exposure to the causative agent, whereas seborrheic dermatitis favors inguinal creases as well as vulvar skin and may also be present on the scalp, ear canals, and face. It is controversial whether atopic dermatitis itself presents in a vulvar location, but atopic patients have a lowered threshold for irritant dermatitis, which has the same appearance as atopic dermatitis.

All types of dermatitis look similar histopathologically, showing spongiosis and varying degrees of epidermal thickening. Although biopsies do not distinguish among the various types of dermatitis, they do help rule out other diseases in the differential diagnosis.

Contact Dermatitis

CD results from exposure to external substances, either irritants or allergens, resulting in inflammation at the site of contact. Irritant CD results from direct damage to keratinocytes without prior sensitization. Allergic CD is a type IV hypersensitivity reaction and requires prior exposure, allowing sensitization to allergens. Although the precise prevalence is not clear, irritant CD is more common than allergic CD. Although CD may be the primary cause of vulvar symptoms, it more commonly arises in the setting of an underlying vulvar disease due to topical products used for treatment or skin care habits.[20]

CD of the vulva should be suspected in patients with pruritus, irritation, or burning and in patients with other vulvar dermatoses not improving with appropriate therapy. Inflamed skin from other diseases predisposes to development of CD by facilitating passage of irritants or allergens into the epidermis.

In allergic CD, sensitized patients classically develop the rash 48 hours after exposure to their allergen. In CD from ongoing allergen exposure, this timing will be less apparent. Women with irritant CD often complain of irritation, rawness and itching, whereas those with allergic CD often have very pronounced degrees of itching.

Patients should be questioned on the use of topical vulvar prescription and over-the-counter products, contraceptives, and hygiene habits. In allergic CD, patients may transfer allergens inadvertently from products used at other sites (**Table 5**). Identifying causative contactants may be difficult, as patients often dismiss them as not being relevant.

CD may be acute, subacute, or chronic. Acute CD manifests as edema, erythema, and occasionally bullae that evolve into weeping erosions. Subacute and CD present with ill-defined scaling erythematous patches and plaques. The scale may be very subtle because of the occluded nature of vulvar skin. Lichenification may be present in long-standing disease. The eruption begins at the site of exposure. Although irritant CD remains localized, allergic CD often spreads locally beyond the site of contact (**Fig. 9**).

A skin biopsy may confirm a diagnosis of dermatitis but does not clearly differentiate allergic from irritant CD. The presence of eosinophils favors a diagnosis of allergic CD; however, they are not always present. Pathology shows spongiosis with psoriasiform

Table 5	
Common vulvar irritants and allergens	
Irritants	**Allergens**
Urine	Topical anesthetics: lidocaine, benzocaine, tetracaine
Feces	Topical antibiotics: neomycin, bacitracin, polymyxin
Sweat	Antifungals: imidazole, nystatin
Abnormal vaginal discharge	Chlorhexidine, thimerosal
Overbathing, excessive hygiene habits	Fragrance
Feminine hygiene products: lubricants, sanitary napkins, feminine hygiene wipes	Preservatives
Hair dryer	Corticosteroids
Soaps and detergents	Lanolin
Medications: alcohol-based creams & gels, propylene glycol, spermicides	Rubber-latex
	Spermicides

Data from Margesson L. Contact dermatitis of the vulva. Dermatol Ther 2004;17(1):20–7; and Schlosser B. Contact dermatitis of the vulva. Dermatol Clin 2010;28(4):697–706.

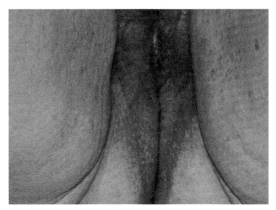

Fig. 9. Subacute CD showing erythema and fine scale.

epidermal hyperplasia in more chronic disease. Biopsies are helpful in ruling out other conditions. Patch testing is essential to identify allergens and is typically performed by dermatologists. Treatment options for contact dermatitis are outlined in **Boxes 1** and **2**.

INFECTIOUS
Candidiasis

Vulvovaginal candidiasis (VVC) is an infection of the vulvovaginal skin caused by the presence of candidal organisms. Infection occurs most often in reproductive-aged women, with greater than 50% of women having experienced VVC sometime in their lifetime. This disorder is less common in females who are estrogen depleted, such as prepubescent girls and postmenopausal women. However, in postmenopausal women using estrogen therapy, VVC should be considered if symptoms are reported. Greater than 90% of infections are caused by *Candida albicans*, with the remaining 10% accounting for atypical *Candida* species, particularly *Candida glabrata*.

Box 1
Pharmacologic treatment options for contact dermatitis

Treat inflammation
    Topical corticosteroids for 3 to 4 weeks
    Ointments preferred
    Betamethasone ointment 0.05% twice a day if severe
    Triamcinolone ointment 0.1% twice a day if moderate
    2.5% Hydrocortisone ointment if mild or for maintenance
    Prednisone 0.5 to 1 mg/kg tapered over 2 to 3 weeks if severe

Treat itching
    Loratadine 10 mg, fexofenadine 60 mg, or cetirizine 10 mg in the morning
    Hydroxyzine 25 to 50 mg every bedtime, doxepin 10 to 25 mg every bedtime (may be sedating)

Prevent or treat infection, if present
    Consider oral fluconazole 150 mg weekly while on corticosteroids for *Candida* suppression
    Oral antibiotics as needed per culture for secondary impetiginization

Adapted from Margesson L. Contact dermatitis of the vulva. Dermatol Ther 2004;17(1):23.

Box 2
Nonpharmacologic treatment options for contact dermatitis

Identify and discontinue irritants and allergens

Lukewarm sitz baths without soap twice a day

Petrolatum or zinc oxide, to create and help restore barrier function

Add estrogen if appropriate

Cool packs to decrease symptoms

Avoid tight clothing and overcleansing

Manage incontinence

Goal to avoid long-term topical corticosteroids: use for flares

Ensure treatment of secondary infection

Review compliance

Women with VVC present with symptoms of vulvar pruritus, burning, irritation, dyspareunia, fissures, and vaginal discharge (**Fig. 10**). Not all women with VVC will report the characteristic white clumpy curdlike discharge that has come to be associated with this infection.

Physical examination should include careful inspection of the vulva for increased erythema, fissures, and edema. Biopsy may be necessary if diagnosis is elusive after examination of the vagina. A speculum examination of the vagina is also necessary to collect swabs for microscopy, vaginal pH (normal 3.5–4.5), and fungal culture. The vaginal pH does not change in VVC. The use of point-of-care polymerase chain reaction (PCR) vaginitis tests is particular to the institution but can provide immediate information as to the presence or absence of *Candida*. Typically, these tests do not identify the species of yeast. However, this is usually only necessary in complicated or recurrent cases of VVC (**Table 6**). Additionally, the ubiquitous use of over-the-counter intravaginal antifungal (azole) medications and over-the-phone prescriptions of oral fluconazole has made it increasingly difficult for clinicians to diagnose VVC. Thus, a fungal culture can be a valuable tool for the clinician when microscopy is not diagnostic (**Box 3**).

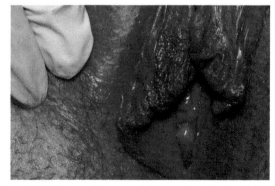

Fig. 10. Candidiasis with bright erythema and fissure of right intralabial sulcus.

Table 6
Features of complicated versus uncomplicated vulvovaginal candidiasis

VVC Features				
Uncomplicated	Sporadic, infrequent <3 episodes per year	Mild to moderate symptoms	Infection with *Candida albicans*	Healthy, nonpregnant woman
Complicated	Severe symptoms	Nonalbicans species of *Candida*	Pregnant, immunocompromised, poorly controlled diabetes	>4 episodes per year

Distinguishing complicated versus uncomplicated VVC is key to choosing the correct treatment in order to obtain symptom control and mycologic cure (see **Table 6**).[8,21,22]

For uncomplicated VVC:

- Use a single-dose 150 mg oral fluconazole.

OR

- Use a 3- to 7-day course of intravaginal azole cream (ie, miconazole, clotrimazole, terconazole).
- Most women prefer the convenience of a single oral tablet over a course of intravaginal cream.

For complicated cases

- Use sequential doses of 150 mg oral fluconazole (2 or 3 doses taken 3 days apart).

OR

- Use a 7- to 14-day course of intravaginal azole cream (ie, miconazole, clotrimazole, terconazole).
- Some women with significant vulvitis may need to be treated with a low-strength steroid ointment (see **Table 4**) for a 3- to 7-day course to reduce the symptoms of inflammation, pruritus, and fissure.

Tinea

Tinea is a dermatophyte infection of the skin that causes superficial skin disease by infecting keratinized tissue, including skin, hair, and nails. It is one of the more common causes of skin infection overall. The clinical types of tinea are defined by their anatomic location, with tinea cruris being a dermatophyte infection of the genital region, groin, and thighs.[23]

Box 3
Tools to evaluate for vulvovaginal candidiasis

- Vaginal pH
- Microscopy with 10% KOH
- Fungal culture
- −/+ Point-of-care vaginitis PCR test
- −/+ Vulvar biopsy

Tinea cruris typically affects adults, occurring much more often in men than women, most commonly caused by *Trichophyton rubrum*. It can be acquired from another infected person or transmitted by fomites after direct skin contact. Predisposing factors include a warm humid environment, atopic diathesis, obesity, tight-fitting clothing, use of topical corticosteroids, or an immunosuppressed status. Tinea cruris tends to be a chronic condition, waxing and waning, with patients often also having tinea pedis, which is thought to be the source of the crural infection. The skin eruption is usually pruritic.

The characteristic lesions are scaling, sharply demarcated, red to tan patches and plaques with a raised advancing border. These lesions typically involve inguinal creases, keratinized vulvar skin in women, and inner thighs but can extend to the buttocks and abdomen if severe. Lesions are often annular with central clearing and may coalesce to form large poly cyclic plaques. The additional presence of papules and pustules indicates follicular involvement. Lichenification can be present secondary to chronic scratching.[23,24]

If misdiagnosed and treated with topical corticosteroids, the characteristic features may be altered making the diagnosis difficult.

Although a diagnosis of tinea may be suspected clinically, a potassium hydroxide (KOH) preparation is recommended to confirm the diagnosis, as other skin diseases may have similar appearance. A fungal culture can also confirm a diagnosis. The culture is obtained from the infected skin not the vagina like vulvovaginal candidiasis.

Most infections can be managed with topical therapy, if no follicular involvement is present. Medications should be applied twice daily for 4 weeks including 1 week after clearing.

Topical therapies include:

- Imidazoles: clotrimazole, miconazole, econazole, ketoconazole
- Allylamines: terbinafine, naftifine

Systemic therapy is usually not needed for tinea cruris; but if there is extensive disease, patients have failed topicals, follicular disease is present, or if patients are immunosuppressed, oral therapy is appropriate. Regimens are similar to what is used for tinea corporis, including:[24]

- Terbinafine 250 mg daily × 1 to 2 weeks
- Itraconazole 200 mg/d × 1 week
- Fluconazole 150 to 200 mg weekly × 2 to 4 weeks
- Griseofulvin microsize 500 to 1000 mg/d × 2 to 4 weeks
- Griseofulvin Ultramicrosize 375 to 500 mg/d × 2 to 4 weeks

Treatment of tinea cruris, pedis, and/or unguium, if present, is important for a good outcome. Reinfection is common and may be minimized by wearing shower shoes in public facilities (or at home if family members are infected), preventive use of topical antifungals 3 times a week, wearing loose clothes, drying well after bathing, weight reduction, laundering contaminated clothing and linens, and use of noncotton underwear.

Perianal Streptococcal Disease

Perianal streptococcal disease is an uncommon form of cutaneous streptococcal infection most often caused by group A beta-hemolytic streptococci. It typically presents as painful perianal erythema and painful defecation but may extend to perineal and vulvar skin. It is most often seen in children, but many adults with this condition have also been described.[25]

Common symptoms include itching, rectal pain, constipation due to pain, blood-streaked stools, painful defecation, and mucoid anal discharge. Pruritus and tenderness are present in vulvar and perineal skin when involved. The disease is frequently misdiagnosed as irritant dermatitis or candidiasis for months, delaying therapy. Intrafamilial spread has been identified in many cases.[26]

Patients present with sharply demarcated, bright erythema perianally; edema and erosions may also be present. The erythema may extend to the perineum and vulva with fissures and scaling.

Patients do not have associated fever or systemic symptoms because of the superficial location of the infection.

Bacterial cultures are necessary to identify group A beta-hemolytic streptococci or other non–group a streptococci occasionally found as the cause.

Oral antibiotic therapy is typically recommended for most patients with penicillin, amoxicillin, or erythromycin for 2 to 3 weeks. Mild cases may be treated with mupirocin 2% ointment 3 times a day for 10 days.[25,26]

Posttreatment culture is important to confirm a cure, as untreated disease can be associated with poststreptococcal glomerulonephritis. Follow-up is advised because recurrence is fairly common. Culturing family members may be of value as they may be carriers.

A urinalysis 1 month after completion of therapy should be considered to rule out poststreptococcal glomerulonephritis.

Erythrasma

Erythrasma is a superficial skin infection caused by the bacteria *Corynebacterium minutissimum*. Erythrasma occurs in healthy adults, particularly ones living in organized institutions like dorms and barracks, but is more common is adults who are obese, diabetic, and immunocompromised under conditions of moisture and occlusion.

Patients typically present with scaly, pruritic, erythematous patches and plaques in interdigital, intertriginous, and genital skin. Commonly in women these plaques and patches are found in the inframammary skin, axilla, umbilicus, and genitals. Diagnosis is based on clinical suspicion; use of Wood lamp, which shows coral fluorescence of involved skin; gram stain from skin scrapings; and negative KOH preparation. Rarely, biopsy is necessary for the elusive case. The differential diagnosis includes psoriasis, tinea, seborrhea, and vulvovaginal candidiasis. Coinfection with a dermatophyte is common.

Treatment includes:

- Topical clindamycin twice a day × 14 to 21 days
- Topical erythromycin twice a day × 14 to 21 days
- Topical fusidic acid twice a day × 14 days
- Oral clarithromycin 1 g × 14 days
- Oral erythromycin 1 g × 14 days

REFERENCES

1. Darragh T, Colgan T, Thomas Cox J, et al. The lower anogenital squamous terminology standardization project for HPV-associated lesions: background and consensus recommendations from the College of American Pathologists and the American Society for Colposcopy and Cervical Pathology. Int J Gynecol Pathol 2013;32:76.
2. Bornstein J, Bogliatto F, Haefner H, et al. Reutter J for the ISSVD terminology committee. Obstet Gynecol 2016;127(2):264.

3. Sideri M, Jones R, Wilkinson E, et al. Squamous vulvar intraepithelial neoplasia: 2004 modified terminology, ISSVD Vulvar Oncology Subcommittee. J Reprod Med 2005;50:807.

4. Neill SM, Lewis FM, Tatnall FM, et al. British Association of Dermatologists. British Association of Dermatologists' guidelines for the management of lichen sclerosus 2010. Br J Dermatol 2010;163(4):672.

5. Del Pino M, Rodriguez-Carunchio L, Ordi J. Pathways of vulvar intraepithelial neoplasia and squamous cell carcinoma. Histopathology 2013;63:161–75.

6. ACOG Committee Opinion No. 509. Management of vulvar intraepithelial neoplasia. Obstet Gynecol 2011;118(5):1192.

7. Maw RD. Treatment of anogenital warts. Dermatol Clin 1998;16(4):829–34.

8. Workowski KA, Bolan GA. Center for disease control and prevention. Sexually transmitted disease treatment guidelines, 2015. MMWR Recomm Rep 2015; 64(RR-03):1–137.

9. Mahto M, Nathan M, O'Mahony C. More than a decade on: review of the use of imiquimod in lower anogenital intraepithelial neoplasia. Int J STD AIDS 2010;21(1):8.

10. van Seters M, van Beurden M, ten Kate FJ, et al. Treatment of vulvar intraepithelial neoplasia with topical imiquimod. N Engl J Med 2008;358(14):1465.

11. Shepherd V, Davidson E, Davies-Humphries J. Extramammary Paget's disease. BJOG 2005;112:273–9.

12. Chanda JJ. Extramammary Paget's disease: prognosis and relationship to internal malignancy. J Am Acad Dermatol 1985;13(6):1009–14.

13. Lam C, Funaro D. Extramammary Paget's disease: summary of current knowledge. Dermatol Clin 2010;28(4):807–26.

14. Van der Linden M. Paget disease of the vulva. Crit Rev Oncol Hematol 2016;101: 60–74.

15. Delport ES. Extramammary Pagets disease of the vulva: an annotated review of the current literature. J Dermatol 2013;54(1):9–21.

16. Itonaga T, Nakayama H, Mitsuru O, et al. Radiotherapy in patients with extramammary Paget's disease-our own experience and review of the literature. Oncol Res Treat 2014;37:18–22.

17. O'Connor WJ, Lim KK, Zalla MJ, et al. Comparison of Mohs micrographic surgery and wide local excision for extramammary Pagets disease. Dermatol Surg 2003; 29(7):723–7.

18. Eczema/dermatitis. In: Wolff K, Johnson R, editors. Fitzpatrick's synopsis of clinical dermatology. 6th edition. New York: McGraw-Hill; 2009. p. 20–52.

19. Crone AM, Stewart EJ, Wojnarowska F, et al. Aetiologic factors in vulvar dermatitis. J Eur Acad Dermatol Venereol 2000;14:181–6.

20. Margesson L. Contact dermatitis of the vulva. Dermatol Ther 2004;17:20–7.

21. Sobel JD. Vulvovaginal candidosis. Lancet 2007;369(9577):1961.

22. Pappas PG, Kauffman CA, Andes D, et al. Clinical practice guidelines for the management of candidiasis: 2009 update by the Infectious Diseases Society of America. Clin Infect Dis 2009;48(5):503.

23. Sobera J, Elewski B. Fungal diseases. In: Bolognia J, editor. Dermatology. 2nd edition. Mosby Elsevier; 2008. p. 1135–49.

24. Kaushik N, Pujalte GG, Reese ST. Superficial fungal infections. Prim Care 2015; 42(4):501–16.

25. Herbst R. Perianal streptococcal disease: recognition. Am J Clin Dermatol 2003; 4(8):555–60.

26. Brilliant LC. Perianal streptococcal dermatitis. Am Fam Physician 2000;61(2): 391–3.

Atopic and Contact Dermatitis of the Vulva

Rita Pichardo-Geisinger, MD

KEYWORDS

- Atopic dermatitis • Eczema • Lichen simplex chronicus • Contact dermatitis
- Irritant dermatitis

KEY POINTS

- Pruritus is a common symptom in a patient with atopic, irritant, or allergic contact dermatitis.
- The diagnosis requires a careful history and physical examination, at times supplemented with a biopsy and/or patch test.
- The 5 most common allergens from the standard series to cause a positive reaction were gold sodium thiosulfate 0.5%, nickel sulfate hexahydrate 2.5%, balsam of Peru 25%, fragrance mix 8%, and cobalt chloride 1%.

Pruritus, or itch, is a common vulvar complaint that is very often treated empirically as a yeast infection; however, yeast infections are just one of the many conditions that can cause vulvar itch. Ignoring these other conditions can do a disservice to your patient by prolonging their pruritus unnecessarily. Atopic dermatitis, irritant contact dermatitis, and allergic contact dermatitis are extremely common noninfectious causes of vulvar itch that are often underdiagnosed by nondermatologists. Up to 50% of cases of chronic vulvovaginal pruritus in adult women can be attributed to irritant and allergic contact dermatitis,[1] and atopic and irritant contact dermatitis are the most common vulvar disorders that present among prepubertal girls, representing one-third of all patients in an Australian series with vulvar disease.[2] Identifying these conditions and treating them appropriately can significantly improve a patient's quality of life and appropriately decrease health care expenditures by preventing unnecessary additional referrals or follow-up visits and decreasing pharmaceutical costs. This article provides an approach to the clinical evaluation and management of these 3 eczematous vulvar disorders.

ATOPIC DERMATITIS

Atopic dermatitis (eczema) is a common, chronic inflammatory skin condition characterized by the presence of red itchy patches and thin plaques on the skin. The development

Disclosure Statement: No conflicts of interest.
Department of Dermatology, Wake Forest University School of Medicine, 4618 Country Club Road, Winston-Salem, NC 27104, USA
E-mail address: rpichard@wakehealth.edu

Obstet Gynecol Clin N Am 44 (2017) 371–378
http://dx.doi.org/10.1016/j.ogc.2017.05.003
0889-8545/17/© 2017 Elsevier Inc. All rights reserved.

of atopic dermatitis results from an interaction between hereditary (genetic) and environmental factors, including a defect in the skin barrier function and changes in the weather making the skin more susceptible to irritation. Some patients have a genetic predisposition for the development of allergic IgE reactions to common environmental allergens, as demonstrated by a personal or family history of allergic rhinitis (hay fever), asthma, and/or atopic dermatitis, otherwise known as the atopic triad.

At the microscopic level, greater transepidermal water loss and thus lower skin surface hydration levels are some of the characteristics of a disrupted skin barrier. Vulvar skin is particularly prone to barrier dysfunction because of irritation caused by sweat, urine and/or feces, the use of irritating and/or allergenic products including baby and adult wipes, washcloths, lubricants, hygiene products, deodorized pads, tampons, overwashing, condoms, tight pants, G-strings, shaving, waxing, or cycling, and sexual encounters that may worsen the primary disease. In addition, the changes in the skin barrier may induce an immune response related to type 2 T helper lymphocytes (Th2 type). Severe pruritus is the most common characteristic of eczema. It may be worse during the evening and exacerbated by sweating or wool clothing. This is at least one of the ways that the itch–scratch cycle starts.

Diagnostic Evaluation

A diagnosis of eczema is made by the combination of a history of itching and scratching along with typical clinical findings. Biopsy may also play a role if the diagnosis cannot be confirmed via history and physical examination findings. Evaluating for infection, especially candidiasis or dermatophytosis, is important because it can mimic eczema. It is also possible to develop a superinfection on top of eczema, because both topical corticosteroid use and the eczema itself are correlated with an increased risk of infection compared with noneczematous vulvar skin.[3]

Atopic dermatitis presents acutely as poorly demarcated erythematous edematous plaques with vesicles, subacutely as erythematous patches or plaques, and chronically as accentuated skin markings or a thickened lichenified plaque.[4] Excoriations may be present secondary to scratching. Repetitive trauma, scratching, or rubbing may lead to postinflammatory pigmentary alteration, either hyperpigmentation or hypopigmentation (**Fig. 1**).

The histologic findings of eczema depend of the stage of the lesion that is biopsied. In an acute lesion, there is a combination of spongiosis, intraepidermal edema with microvesiculation or macrovesiculation and inflammatory infiltrates composed of lymphocytes, eosinophils, and mast cells in the upper dermis. In an older lesion, spongiosis persists, but vesiculation tends to dissipate. As the lesion progresses in chronicity, the epidermis gets progressively thicker owing to hyperplasia (called acanthosis) and inflammation and spongiosis may become mild or absent.

Management

Patient counseling regarding the chronic nature of atopic dermatitis and its management is critical. Patient education is fundamental to achieve control of this disease. It is important for patients to understand that control, rather than cure, is the goal.

The management of atopic dermatitis can be fundamentally characterized by 4 factors:

- Eliminating irritant and allergen exposure,
- Controlling pruritus,
- Repairing barrier function, and
- Applying topical antiinflammatory agents.

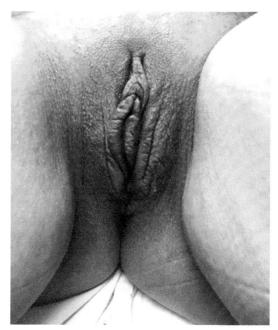

Fig. 1. Vulvar atopic dermatitis in a patient with history of atopic dermatitis.

Eliminating irritant and allergen exposure

Avoiding and eliminating exposure to irritants, especially overwashing, lubricants, topical hygiene products, panty liners, deodorized pads, urine, feces, and excessive perspiration, is important. It is strongly recommended that women use a fragrance-free bar of soap for cleansing. Bubble baths, salts, and oils may irritate the vulvar skin and should be avoided. Addressing mechanical irritation can be critical for some patients, who may be scrubbing with loofahs, towels, and even steel wool! Pointing out the skin damage that these physical irritants may be causing is the first step to modifying behavior.

Similarly, avoiding and eliminating exposure to allergens is also critical. Common allergens to avoid will be addressed elsewhere in this article.

Controlling pruritus

Control of the pruritus, especially during the night, with sedating H1 antihistaminic agents such as hydroxyzine can help to break the itch–scratch cycle. Hydroxyzine is recommended in doses of 10 to 25 mg/d. The most common side effects are dizziness and drowsiness; for this reason, we recommend this medication at bedtime. Another alternative is doxepin, a trycyclic antidepressant, in doses of 10 to 30 mg at bedtime. Drowsiness, dry mouth, and dizziness are the most common side effects of this medication. It is recommended to not use doxepin if the patient has an untreated narrow angle glaucoma or severe trouble urinating. Also this medication should not be used if the patient is taking a monoamine oxidase inhibitor.

Repairing barrier function

Skin barrier dysfunction may produce dry, flaky, itchy skin, which aggravates atopic dermatitis. It may be improved with the appropriate use of petroleum jelly, dimethicone, or zinc oxide paste 2 or 3 times a day.

Applying topical antiinflammatories

Topical antiinflammatory medication is a cornerstone to the treatment of eczema. The more lichenification or epidermal thickening that is present on examination, the higher the potency of topical corticosteroids that will be needed to control disease. Please refer to the article on lichen simplex chronicus in this journal issue for further details. When lichenification is not present, a mild to moderate strength topical corticosteroid is often sufficient, for example, triamcinolone 0.1% ointment. Once the pruritus and physical examination findings are improved, the frequency of use can be tapered or the medicine can be substituted for a lower potency topical corticosteroids. Topical calcineurin inhibitors such as tacrolimus (Protopic) ointment or pimecrolimus (Elidel) cream can be helpful as adjunctive or even primary treatment, especially when steroid atrophy is present on examination.[5]

If a patient does not improve after this management plan is implemented, a biopsy should be seriously considered, especially to rule out an alternative diagnosis such as malignancy. In certain cases, it may be helpful to have your surgical pathology specimen also reviewed by a dermatopathologist, especially if the pathology read is inconsistent with your clinical diagnosis.

IRRITANT AND ALLERGIC CONTACT DERMATITIS
Definitions

Contact dermatitis is an inflammatory disorder caused by exposure to an external agent that acts as either a direct irritant (irritant contact dermatitis) or as an antigen prompting an immunologic reaction (allergic contact dermatitis). Both types of contact dermatitis are common in adults. In contrast, irritant contact dermatitis is common in children wearing diapers, whereas allergic contact dermatitis is infrequent in this population.[2] Burning or irritation is more commonly associated with an irritant contact dermatitis and itch is more commonly associated with an allergic contact dermatitis, although there can be overlap in symptom presentation.

Irritant contact dermatitis results from a local toxic effect from application of an irritant to the skin. One hundred percent of people exposed to a specific irritant would eventually develop contact dermatitis if sufficient quantity was applied.

In contrast, allergic contact dermatitis is a type IV or delayed-type hypersensitivity reaction in which the skin is reexposed to an antigen to which the patient has previously been sensitized. Only a small portion of people exposed to a specific allergen will actually develop sensitization over time. Factors that influence the risk of sensitization include the chemical structure of the allergen, an individual's genetic predisposition, age, preexisting tissue injury, and other factors.[6] Whereas irritant contact dermatitis evolves very rapidly, within minutes to a few hours, the allergic form takes longer to develop, usually 24 to 48 hours. Marren and colleagues[7] studied the correlation between patch tests results of 135 patients presenting with vulvar symptoms. Of them, 63 patients (47%) had at least 1 positive reaction. Relevant hypersensitivity was found related to ethylenediamine, neomycin, framycetin, and clobetasol propionate.

The Vulva as a High-Risk Site

There is scientific evidence indicating that vulvar skin demonstrates more reactivity to chemical irritants than exposed skin.[8,9] The vulva can be considered analogous to the lower legs in a patient with venous stasis; both sites are at increased risk of contact allergen sensitization owing to the frequent use of multiple medicaments in the area. Additionally, the vulva is a site of potential friction from sexual activity; maceration from body secretions such as urine, feces, and vaginal discharge; and low estrogen, which all degrade barrier function.[10,11] Iatrogenic causes of irritant contact dermatitis include trichloroacetic acid, fluorouracil, podofilox gel, and imiquimod and even abortifactents.[12–15]

Irritants and allergens abound in over-the-counter products used on the vulva. More than one-half of 114 postmenopausal women questioned in a recent cross-sectional study used at least 1 over-the-counter product in the last 3 months with one-third of the women having used 2 or more products.[16] High-risk products include topical benzocaine cream, sanitary napkins,[17,18] and baby wipes,[19] to name a few.

In dermatology, we have witnessed an increasing preference for the use of botanic products owing to the belief by patients that these compounds are more natural and safer, in comparison with the synthetic ones. In a study of 66 patients, Corazza and colleagues[20] reported that 63.6% used natural products, 16.7% reported the use on regular basis; 71 different herbal products were identified by patients. The products that contained botanic compounds were creams, vaginal suppositories and vaginal plugs, and perfumes and deodorants. The botanic products most commonly used by the patients were chamomile, aloe vera, *Calendula officinalis*, and *Arnica montana*. A total of 16.7% of patients reported side effects resulting in worsening of the preexisting dermatitis or symptoms of itching, burning, erythema, swelling, and vesiculation. All of the patients underwent patch testing with the SIDAPA and the supplementary series. The most common allergens that were positive in the SIDAPA series were nickel sulfate, fragrance mix I, *Myroxylon pereirae*, methylchloroisothiazolinone/methylisothiazolinone and fragrance mix II. Two patients had reactions to topical corticosteroids that were considered clinically significant.[20]

More evidence is accumulating regarding the association between ingestion of certain irritants and allergens and vulvovaginal symptoms. Examples include nickel dietary intake in patients with nickel allergy; food preservatives, additives, and dyes; and fragrances such as peppermint tea.[21] This highlights the detective work that is sometimes needed to help identify the culprit allergen for refractory cases of contact dermatitis.

O'Gorman and Torgerson[22] studied 90 patients who were tested to allergens in the standard (most common and important allergens in North America) and gynecologic series, the authors found 62 patients (69%) had at least 1 positive result. Forty-one of these patients (46%) had multiple positive results. The 5 most common allergens from the standard series to cause a positive reaction were gold sodium thiosulfate 0.5%, nickel sulfate hexahydrate 2.5%, balsam of Peru 25%, fragrance mix 8%, and cobalt chloride 1%. There were 21 reactions to allergens from the gynecologic series; these included terconazole cream 0.8%, benzoic acid 5%, and paraben mix 16%. In addition, reactions occurred in relation to propylene glycol 10%, clindamycin phosphate 2%, clotrimazole 1%, tioconazole, conjugate estrogen 0.625 mg/g, and sodium lauryl sulfate 0.1% aqueous. Positive reactions to steroids such as tixocortol-21-pivalat 1% were also observed. The most common antibiotic allergen found was neomycin sulfate 20%, and terconazole was the most common antifungal in this series. Benzocaine was also tested and it caused a positive response in most of the patients.[22] It is important to consider the cross-reaction between benzocaine and sulfa drugs, para-aminobenzoic acid and paraphenylenediamine, in patients with history of sulfa allergy or a hair dye allergy and vulvar disease.[23]

Diagnostic Evaluation

A medical evaluation of contact dermatitis requires

1. A complete clinical history including a questionnaire completed by the patient before seeing the physician (if possible); this can be very helpful to identify the

products (over-the-counter and by prescription) that the patient uses, the symptoms and their severity and the timeline and association with the development of the clinical findings,[4]
2. A high level of suspicion for a possible irritant and/or allergen, and
3. The ability to perform and interpret an appropriate patch test result if allergic contact dermatitis is suspected.

On physical examination, it can be challenging to distinguish allergic contact dermatitis from irritant contact dermatitis and atopic dermatitis, especially in their chronic forms. It is recommended to assume that an irritant component is present in all eczematous vulvar conditions, with or without allergens.[11] Intermittent symptoms may be a clue for the diagnosis of allergic contact dermatitis.[23] A diagnosis of allergic contact dermatitis should be suspected in patients who apply multiple agents to their skin and whose pruritus does not respond to usual therapy.[4] Significant pruritus would favor a diagnosis of atopic or allergic contact dermatitis over pure irritant contact dermatitis, which tends to cause more burning or irritation. The characteristic clinical findings in contact dermatitis are a well-demarcated erythematous vesicular plaque or a scaly patch corresponding to the area of contact (**Fig. 2**).

A biopsy may be helpful to exclude other pathologies if a diagnosis cannot be achieved based on history and physical examination alone. The histopathology of allergic contact dermatitis is most useful in acute lesions, where microscopic findings include spongiosis, and a mixed inflammatory dermal infiltrate composed of lymphocytes, histiocytes, and a variable number of eosinophils. In severe reactions, vesiculation is also present. Chronic processes are largely characterized by psoriasiform epidermal hyperplasia (otherwise known as acanthosis).

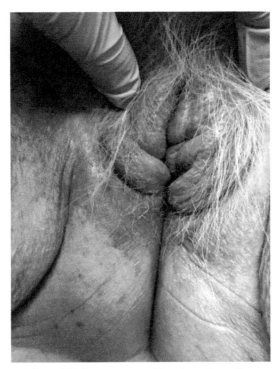

Fig. 2. Irritant contact dermatitis in a woman with urinary incontinence.

Owing to the similar and overlapping clinical and pathologic features of these 2 entities, patch testing can be a useful tool to help identify a specific contact allergen. The patch test is the gold standard for the diagnoses of allergic contact dermatitis. Patch testing is a time-consuming office procedure that requires well-trained personnel and is poorly reimbursed. Patients should be referred to a dermatologist who performs patch testing. This type of testing is very different from the type 1 allergy testing performed by Allergy and Immunology specialists. The TRUE test, which is approved by the US Food and Drug Administration, is a commercially available standard patch test that screens for 35 allergens and 1 negative control spot. Most general dermatologists perform this form of patch testing. The TRUE test can be helpful when positive but many relevant allergens in our vulvar patients are not present in this limited series; thus, a negative test does not rule out allergic contact dermatitis in your patient. It is important to refer a patient with suspected allergic contact dermatitis and a negative TRUE test to a dermatologist who specializes in contact dermatitis and patch testing. Expanded series testing can then be performed by this subspecialized expert.

Management

As in atopic dermatitis, patient education is critical in the management of contact dermatitis. Any component of urinary or fecal incontinence should be managed aggressively. Patients need to understand how to read product labels and become proactive in identifying possible irritants and allergens in the products they are using, because identifying and avoiding the culprit irritant(s) and allergen(s) is critical to achieving disease control. Otherwise, the management of contact dermatitis is almost identical to the management of atopic dermatitis reviewed earlier in this article, which is not repeated here. In severe cases of acute contact dermatitis, a short course of systemic steroids such as oral prednisone may be needed, which is much less commonly warranted for atopic dermatitis.

SUMMARY

Irritant and atopic dermatitis are the most common dermatoses of the vulva in children and adults. Allergic contact dermatitis is common in adult women, but it is uncommon in children. Symptoms of burning and pruritus should alert the physician to the possibility of these conditions. A careful history and good examination will identify most cases. In a minority of individuals, other testing such as skin biopsy or patch testing may help to confirm a diagnosis. Once a diagnosis has been established, irritant and allergenic products should be avoided and an appropriate vulvar care regimen should be implemented. A multipronged approach to management of these eczematous conditions should enable good disease control, thus improving the quality of life of your patients with vulvar pruritus and irritation.

REFERENCES

1. Farage MA, Miller KW, Ledger WJ. Determining the cause of vulvovaginal symptoms. Obstet Gynecol Surv 2008;63(7):445–64.
2. Fischer G, Rogers M. Vulvar disease in children: a clinical audit of 130 cases. Pediatr Dermatol 2000;17(1):1–6.
3. Edwards L, Lynch P. 2nd edition. Genital dermatology atlas, 4. Philadelphia: Lippincott Williams & Wilkins; 2011. p. 31–45.
4. Stewart K. Vulvar dermatoses: a practical approach to evaluation and management. JCOM 2012;19(5):205–20.

5. Ho VC, Gupta A, Kaufman R, et al. Safety and efficacy of nonsteroid pimecrolimus cream 1% in the treatment of atopic dermatitis in infants. J Pediatr 2003; 142:155–62.
6. Kamarashev JA, Vassileva SG. Dermatologic diseases of the vulva. Clin Dermatol 1997;15:53–65.
7. Marren P, Wojnarowska F, Powel S. Allergic contact dermatitis and vulvar dermatosis. Br J Dermatol 1992;126:52–6.
8. Britz MB, Maibach HI. Human cutaneous vulvar reactivity to irritants. Contact Dermatitis 1979;5:375–7.
9. Elsner P, Wilhelm D, Maibach HI. The effect of low-concentration sodium lauryl sulfate on human vulvar and forearm skin: age related differences. J Reprod Med 1990;36:77–81.
10. Bauer A, Rödiger C, Greif C, et al. Vulvar dermatosis-irritant and allergic contact dermatitis of the vulva. Dermatology 2005;210:143–9.
11. Margesson LJ. Contact dermatitis of the vulva. Dermatol Ther 2004;17:20–7.
12. Shull JC. Vaginal bleeding from potassium permanganate burns. Am J Obstet Gynecol 1941;41:161.
13. Vandergriff W, Diddle AW. Intravaginal use of potassium permanganate as an abortifacient: the error in diagnosis. Obstet Gynecol 1966;28:155.
14. Beutner KR, Spruance SL, Hougham AJ, et al. Treatment of genital warts with an immune-response modifier (imiquimod). J Am Acad Dermatol 1998;38:230–9.
15. Tyring S, Edwards L, Cherry LK, et al. Safety and efficacy of 0.5% podofilox gel in the treatment of anogenital warts. Arch Dermatol 1998;134:33–8.
16. Erekson EA, Martin DK, Brousseau EC, et al. Over-the-counter treatments and perineal hygiene in postmenopausal women. Menopause 2014;21(3):281–5.
17. Eason EL, Feldman P. Contact dermatitis associated with the use of always sanitary napkins. Can Med Assoc J 1996;154(8):1173–6.
18. Fujimura T, Sato N, Takagi Y, et al. An investigator blinded cross-over study to characterize the cutaneous effects and suitability of modern sanitary pads for menstrual protection for women residing in the USA. Cutan Ocul Toxicol 2011; 30(3):205–11.
19. Foote CA, Brady SP, Brady KL, et al. Vulvar dermatitis from allergy to moist flushable wipes. J Low Genit Tract Dis 2014;18(1):E16–8.
20. Corazza M, Virgili A, Toni G, et al. Level of use and safety of botanical products for itching vulvar dermatosis. Are patch tests useful? Contact Dermatitis 2016;74: 289–94.
21. Vermaat H, van Meurs T, Rustemeyer T, et al. Vulvar allergic contact dermatitis due to peppermint oil in herbal tea. Contact Dermatitis 2008;58:364–5.
22. O'Gorman SM, Torgerson RR. Allergic contact dermatitis of the vulva. Dermatitis 2013;24(2):64–72.
23. Pincus SH. Vulvar dermatosis and pruritus vulvae. Dermatol Clin 1992;10: 297–308.

Vulvar Pruritus and Lichen Simplex Chronicus

Rebecca Chibnall, MD

KEYWORDS

- Vulvar pruritus • Vulvar itch • Lichen simplex chronicus
- Hyperplastic vulvar dystrophy • Squamous cell hyperplasia

KEY POINTS

- Pruritus of the vulva is a common condition with multifactorial cause in girls and women.
- Without treatment with anti-inflammatories, behavioral modification, and symptomatic management, it can lead to the inflammatory dermatitis lichen simplex chronicus.
- These conditions can lead to psychosocial stress and impair work, sleep, and sexual function.
- Remission is attainable with a comprehensive treatment regimen.

INTRODUCTION: NATURE OF THE PROBLEM

Vulvar pruritus and itch is a common complaint among girls and women presenting to gynecologists and dermatologists. Cause of itch, and specifically vulvar itch, is multifactorial and poorly understood. The cellular mechanisms that lead to a sensation of itching have been understudied and misunderstood in the past; however, recently, researchers have been discovering molecular pathways and immune dysregulation that can explain why some people itch.[1] Vulvar itch is even less studied at an epidemiologic and especially molecular level compared with other types of itching, it is complicated by the unique topography of the vulva. The modified mucosal epithelium, combined with the humidity, and many skin folds of the vulva, result in an atypical appearance to rashes that are otherwise easily diagnosed on the rest of the skin. This unique architecture is further complicated because the vulva joins the urinary, reproductive, and digestive tracts, which introduce further potential for irritants. For many patients with vulvar pruritus, an inciting event such as an infectious vulvovaginitis may initiate an itch-scratch cycle that is then perpetuated and complicated by various over-the-counter remedies. In some women, this chronic and untreated itch can lead to the inflammatory dermatitis lichen simplex chronicus (LSC) which further perpetuates the itch-scratch cycle. Left untreated or undertreated, vulvar pruritus and LSC can cause

Disclosure Statement: The author has nothing to disclose.
Department of Dermatology, Washington University School of Medicine, 5201 Midamerica Plaza, Suite 2300, St Louis, MO 63129, USA
E-mail address: rchibnall@wustl.edu

Obstet Gynecol Clin N Am 44 (2017) 379–388
http://dx.doi.org/10.1016/j.ogc.2017.04.003
0889-8545/17/© 2017 Elsevier Inc. All rights reserved.

obgyn.theclinics.com

significant morbidity. Common complaints of women with chronic vulvar itch and LSC include interruption of work, sleep, sexual function, and general discomfort. Herein, an overview of vulvar itch and LSC, including causes (**Table 1**), patient history, physical examination, diagnostic work up, treatment, and follow-up, are discussed.

HISTORY

Women presenting with vulvar itch and LSC primarily complain of itch that is constant or intermittent and feels better with rubbing or scratching.[2] Duration of symptoms and the desire to scratch are both key pieces of information to obtain at the onset of the patient encounter. These women often complain of burning with urination, defecation, and sexual activity secondary to the excoriations produced by chronic scratching. In addition to causing discomfort, these breaks in the barrier can predispose to a variety of nonsexually acquired and sexually acquired infections.[3] Furthermore, disruption of

Table 1 Causes of vulvar pruritus	
Inflammatory	• Lichen sclerosus • Lichen planus • Plasma cell vulvitis • Psoriasis
Neoplastic	• Differentiated vulvar intraepithelial neoplasia and squamous cell carcinoma • Verrucous carcinoma • Extramammary Paget disease • Syringomas
Infections	• Candidiasis • Bacterial vaginosis • Dermatophytosis
Infestations	• Pediculosis pubis and corporis • Scabies • Enterobiasis (mostly seen in children)

Environmental	• Irritant contact dermatitis
	  ○ Leukorrhea in desquamative inflammatory vaginitis
	  ○ Urine
	  ○ Feces
	  ○ Condoms
	  ○ Lubricants
	  ○ Menstrual and incontinence pads
	  ○ Tampons
	  ○ Foreign body
	• Allergic contact dermatitis
	  ○ Topical anesthetics
	  ○ Fragrance
	  ○ Preservatives
	  ○ Rubber allergens
	  ○ Spermicides
	  ○ Corticosteroids

Neuropathic	• Postherpetic pruritus • Diabetic neuropathy • Lumbosacral arthritis • Spine injuries or surgeries
Hormonal	• Atrophic vaginitis

sleep, especially inability to fall asleep due to the desire to scratch, is a common complaint. As such, women suffering from vulvar itch experience further complications secondary and tertiary to the actual itch. Quality of life surveys have been done for several other conditions that produce chronic itch, including hemodialysis patients. These studies all support that with worsening and chronicity of itch, the patient's quality of life suffers accordingly.[4] Moreover, the culturally sensitive nature of the vulva makes vulvar pruritus especially disruptive. A woman's desire to scratch can lead to disruption at work and inability to have comfortable sexual relations.

Many women identify that their pruritus symptoms began with a specific trigger, often a self-diagnosed yeast infection, or other vaginitis. When obtaining history in a patient with vulvar pruritus, a thorough review of the patient's vulvar care regimen is essential to ruling out superimposed irritant or allergic contact dermatitis (ACD). In recent years, at-home vaginal health test kits have become commonplace in pharmacies across the country. In store aisles, women are bombarded with marketing for products that are termed refreshing, cleansing, and promise instant relief from itching.[5] Common ingredients that cause ACD in these products include the anesthetic benzocaine, fragrance, and preservatives, such as the 2013 American Contact Dermatitis Society Allergen of the year, methylisothiazolinone.[6] Many women will attempt self-treatment of their pruritus with these over-the-counter remedies and thereby complicate their condition with an ACD. Moreover, condoms, douches, lubricants, spermicides, soaps, disposable pads, and tampons are often culprits in irritant contact dermatitis.[2] With the ubiquity of these products and their advertised relief for itching and other vaginal or vulvar irritations, women continue to self-treat their vulvar itch, exacerbating the underlying condition. Due to societal stigmatization regarding vaginal and vulvar issues, women frequently fail to seek appropriate dermatologic or gynecologic treatment from a physician. Thus, what may appear to the patient as a yeast infection will be treated as such, only to compound the patient's issue and lead to further exacerbation of her pruritus.

Additionally, it is important to recognize that vulvar pruritus and LSC often occur in the setting of other vulvar dermatoses. The patient's past dermatologic history should be reviewed. Prior diagnoses of eczema, psoriasis, and oral or cutaneous lichen planus (LP) can be extremely helpful in pinpointing the cause of vulvar symptoms. This in conjunction with the physical examination may identify an inflammatory process compounded by pruritus and LSC.

Furthermore, gynecologic history, including prior abnormal pap smears; reproductive tract malignancy; and, if relevant, age at menopause, can assist in identifying if a malignancy or state of atrophy could be the cause of the pruritus. Medication history containing details of any hormone replacement therapy is essential because women on oral contraceptives or estrogen are unlikely to have atrophic vaginitis. History should also include whether or not any household members or sexual partners are experiencing pruritus because this can suggest an infection or infestation.

Finally, ascertaining any history of atopy, arthritis, spine surgeries or injuries, zoster infections, and diabetes can be helpful in identifying patients with atopic itch or neuropathic itch. Differentiating these conditions can direct oral anti-itch therapy toward either histamine blockade or neuropathic-targeted treatment. These pearls of information are all useful in stressing gentle vulvar care and directing itch treatment.

PHYSICAL EXAMINATION

The keratinized vulva in vulvar pruritus and LSC demonstrates red and/or hyperpigmented plaques with increased skin markings and a varying degree of scale. The medial thighs may also display red and/or hyperpigmented scaly and lichenified plaques. Prurigo or picker's nodules may be present on the keratinized skin in severe cases. Occasionally, hypopigmented or white and sometimes atrophic scars may be present in patients who have scratched severely. Because of the moist nature of the vulva relative to nongenital skin, scale often appears as white plaques with maceration. In addition, excoriations as well as broken hairs are common (**Fig. 1**). Nonkeratinized skin medial to Hart's lines often appears primarily erythematous and/or hyperpigmented, sometimes with thickening. When asked to identify precisely where the primary symptoms are occurring, women may demonstrate scratching behavior.

Additionally, speculum examination and wet mount should be performed to rule out vaginal conditions such as desquamative inflammatory vaginitis (DIV) and atrophic vaginitis. The relatively basic pH and discharge in DIV can cause a pruritic irritant contact dermatitis leading to LSC. This pruritus is unlikely to clear without treatment of the underlying DIV. In DIV, wet mount will display pH greater than 4.5, sheets of white blood cells, parabasal cells, and lack of lactobacilli. Furthermore, loss of mucosal integrity and relative dehydration of the tissue in atrophic vaginitis can also contribute to itch. In this condition, wet mount will show pH greater than 4.5, numerous parabasal cells, few white blood cells, and lack of lactobacilli.[7] In isolated idiopathic vulvar pruritus and LSC, the vagina should be normal in appearance with pink, moist, rugated mucosa.

It is vital to carefully examine the entire skin and obtain a thorough history to rule out inflammatory dermatoses, such as eczema, psoriasis, LP, and lichen sclerosus (LS). Clues on the remaining skin may lead the diagnosis toward one condition over another. Patients with atopic dermatitis or eczema will often have thin pink scaly plaques of the flexures. These patients may also present with hyperlinearity of the palms and periorbitally, and history of atopy may verify this diagnosis. Moreover, a careful investigation for the characteristic red, well-demarcated plaques with silver scale located on the scalp, elbows, knees, umbilicus, and buttocks, as well as the nails for pitting, is often helpful to rule out psoriasis. The gluteal cleft will often be involved in vulvar psoriasis. Because psoriatic plaques can be thick and scale takes on an unusual appearance in the vulva, it is often difficult to distinguish psoriasis from LSC. Close examination of the vulva and vagina for scarring, labial agglutination, reticulate rash, and erosions is also helpful to rule out LP. Oral examination for Wickham striae, which appear as lacy white patches on the buccal mucosa, and skin examination for the characteristic flat-topped, polygonal, and purple plaques of LP can clinch the diagnosis. Finally, hypopigmentation, atrophy, petechiae and purpura, labial

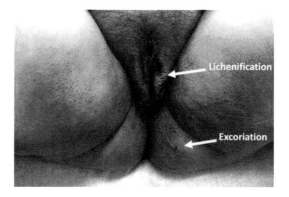

Fig. 1. LSC.

agglutination, and scarring with a figure-of-8 pattern can suggest an underlying LS. These diagnoses can cause such severe pruritus that a subsequent LSC may occur, but care not to miss LS and LP is paramount because they both can lead to severe scarring and increase the risk for differentiated vulvar intraepithelial neoplasia (VIN) and squamous cell carcinoma (SCC).

Furthermore, both benign and malignant tumors of the vulva can cause symptoms of pruritus. Malignancies such as differentiated VIN occur in settings of inflammatory dermatoses. When signs of LS or LP are present, as previously described, any area of the vulva causing particular pain or pruritus should be closely examined for focused erythema, loss of follicular ostia, or absence of skin markings. These lesions should be biopsied, especially if they are refractory to anti-inflammatory therapy. Verrucous carcinoma and invasive SCC of the vulva have also been reported to cause pruritus.[8] Condyloma that appear larger, variably pigmented, or otherwise different than typical condyloma, or are unresponsive to treatment should be biopsied to rule out these 2 conditions. Benign tumors such as syringomas have also been reported to cause pruritus.[9] These growths appear as skin-colored, pink, or hyperpigmented 2 to 4 mm papules primarily on the nonglabrous skin of the vulva. Biopsy for standard pathologic testing confirms the diagnosis and treatment is mostly directed either at destruction via laser or symptomatic treatment.

With environmental, infectious, and infestation causes of vulvar pruritus, lichenification and excoriation may be the primary finding. In ACD, characteristic edematous pink variably scaling plaques may be observed in the areas surrounding lichenification. In acute and severe cases of ACD, edema may be so significant as to cause blistering, and patterned or asymmetrical rash may also be present. These findings, corroborated with history of using implicated agents, should suggest ACD as the cause. Infections such as vulvovaginal candidiasis or bacterial vaginosis should have accompanying vaginal discharge or odor. Still, in the absence of discharge, a wet mount should always be performed to examine for hyphae and/or clue cells because simple erythema and pruritus can still be the presenting sign.[7] Infestations, such as crab lice, body lice, and scabies, must be ruled out in cases of severe pruritus, especially when other household members or sexual partners are affected. Crab lice are often isolated at the base of the pubic hair shaft and can be mistaken for scabbing secondary to excoriation. Unlike crab lice, body lice live in clothing, so excoriations and red papules and macules may be seen on the vulva but clothing should also be examined for eggs and adult louse forms. Finally, scabies is a common cause of pruritus and vulvar pruritus. Scabies most often will be accompanied by pink edematous scaling and crusted papules, occasionally with burrows in the web spaces of the hands and feet, on the volar wrists, in the axilla, inframammary creases, umbilicus, waistline, and ankles.

DIAGNOSIS
Skin Scraping

If scabies or dermatophytosis is suspected, a skin scraping with potassium hydroxide prep can demonstrate the scabies mite, scabies feces (scybala), or eggs. Dermatophytes can also be observed through yeast forms or hyphae seen crossing cell membranes.

Wet Mount

Wet mount should be performed during speculum examination. In vulvar pruritus and LSC, the wet mount should be normal with pH in the range of 3.8 to 4.5, presence of lactobacilli, normal squamous epithelium with minimal to no parabasal cells, no clue cells, no hyphae or yeast forms, and a no greater than 1:1 white blood cell to epithelial cell ratio (**Fig. 2**).[7] Treatment of any abnormality should be completed before diagnosing primary idiopathic vulvar pruritus and LSC.

Skin Biopsy

Biopsy for pathologic testing with hematoxylin-eosin and/or immunofluorescence is usually not necessary for vulvar pruritus and LSC; however, if there is any clinical concern for a primary inflammatory vulvitis, ACD, or benign or malignant neoplasm, tissue pathologic testing may be warranted. Pathologic testing of LSC shows psoriasiform hyperplasia, compact orthokeratosis, and hypergranulosis with no atypia of the epithelial cells.[10]

TREATMENT

Skin-directed therapy for inflammatory and primary vulvar pruritus and LSC should begin with topical corticosteroids. High-potency class 1 topical steroids should be used in severe cases. These are often necessary for a few weeks to a few months used daily or twice a day, then tapered to only a few times a week as needed for symptom recurrence. Side effects of high-potency topical steroids include steroid-induced erythema, striae, and hypopigmentation. When used correctly, the risk of side effects on the modified mucosa of the vulva is low. Ointments should be selected instead of creams and lotions because they are less likely to cause stinging on contact and they are more potent. Clobetasol propionate 0.05% ointment has been the most commonly used high-potency steroid in the past but many patients in the last 2 years have found this medication to be too expensive.[11] Other class 1 steroid options include betamethasone dipropionate 0.05% augmented ointment or halobetasol propionate 0.05% ointment. As the condition improves, or if long-term therapy is anticipated, class 4

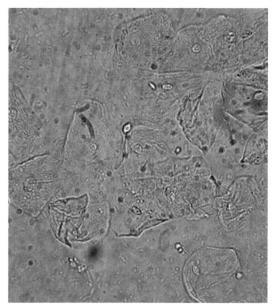

Fig. 2. Normal wet mount.

triamcinolone acetonide 0.1% ointment can be used daily. With topical steroid usage, it should be stressed that a very small amount (less than a pea-size) is adequate for application. Demonstrating where exactly medication should be applied with the use of a handheld mirror can improve compliance. Steroid-sparing agents, such as tacrolimus 0.1% ointment daily, can be used as well. If LSC plaques are very thick and response to high-potency topical steroids is not as expected, injection with intralesional triamcinolone (ILK) into the thickest plaques can be performed in the office. Triamcinolone acetonide 10 mg/cc is injected using a 1 cc Luer locking syringe with 30-gauge one-half inch needle and is tolerated well by patients. If inflammation is severe and there are many excoriations, yeast prophylaxis with fluconazole 150 mg or 200 mg weekly should be considered while on anti-inflammatory therapy.

For symptomatic management, lidocaine 2% jelly applied 15 to 30 minutes before intercourse or ILK injections can be beneficial for topical anesthesia. In patients with an atopic diathesis, nonsedating antihistamines such as cetirizine and fexofenadine dosed twice daily, as well as sedating antihistamines such as diphenhydramine and hydroxyzine every 6 hours as needed for itching, can reduce pruritus and improve sleep. For patients unresponsive to antihistamines, neuromodulators of itch such as amitriptyline and gabapentin can be used. These are usually dosed starting at night secondary to drowsiness. With gabapentin, as patients develop tolerance, the medication can be used for itching relief throughout the day by 3 times a day dosing (**Table 2**).

Nonpharmacologic Treatment Options

Eliminating sources of irritant dermatitis or ACD is essential to resolving vulvar pruritus and LSC. All harsh soaps and cleansers should be discontinued and patients should

Table 2
Pharmacologic treatment of inflammatory and primary vulvar pruritus and lichen simplex chronicus

Treatment of inflammation	
Anti-inflammatory	• Clobetasol propionate 0.05% ointment daily or bid • Betamethasone dipropionate 0.05% augmented ointment daily or bid • Halobetasol propionate 0.05% ointment daily or bid • Triamcinolone 0.1% ointment daily or bid • Tacrolimus 0.1% ointment daily or bid • ILK 10 mg/cc to areas with severe lichenification done q 4–6 wk
Antifungal prophylaxis while using steroids (if inflammation is severe)	• Fluconazole 150 mg or 200 mg po q week
Symptomatic management	
Anesthetic	• Lidocaine 2% jelly applied 15–30 min before intercourse
Nonsedating antihistamine	• Cetirizine 10 mg bid • Fexofenadine 180 mg bid
Sedating antihistamine	• Diphenhydramine 25–50 mg q 6 h prn • Hydroxyzine 10–30 mg q 6 h prn
Neuromodulators	• Amitriptyline 20–30 mg nightly • Gabapentin 300–900 mg nightly for sleep or up to 1200 mg tid for neuropathic itch

be instructed to wash only with water. No wash cloths or loofahs should be used, only gentle cleansing with hands. Douching and feminine washes should be discouraged because they contain many of the irritants and allergens previously discussed. All over-the-counter topical medications should be stopped and only prescribed oint-ments or petroleum jelly should be applied. Frequent emollients with petroleum jelly can alleviate symptoms of LSC throughout the day. Advising patients to keep a tub of petrolatum in the refrigerator at home and a small tube in her purse can provide further relief. Grooming practices, such as shaving, waxing, plucking, and clipping, should be minimized. Menstruating women should consider using silicone menstrual cups (**Fig. 3**) and reusable cloth pads (**Fig. 4**) rather than tampons and pads. Women who require daily use of pads because of urinary or fecal incontinence should use reusable pads or liners instead and change these frequently. Some reusable pads are stay-dry and provide the added benefit of wicking moisture away through a poly-ester fleece material. Lubricants during sexual activity should be limited to vegetable oil, or, if water-based lubricant is necessary, Astroglide should be chosen because others can cause further irritation.[2] Intermittent icing can be beneficial as well; how-ever, patients should be cautioned to apply ice for maximum of 15 minutes at a time due to risk of cold injury.

Combination Therapies

Identification of the cause of vulvar pruritus must come first, then a combination of anti-inflammatory, antineoplastic, or anti-infectious treatment with symptomatic man-agement treatment is usually necessary to control vulvar pruritus and LSC. Patients should be warned that treatments take time and that improvement rarely occurs over-night but rather within weeks to months. Behavioral modification with cutting nails short and encouraging cognizance of scratching is also beneficial. Occasionally, behavioral modification techniques such as cognitive behavioral therapy may be necessary in patients with a deeply rooted itch-scratch cycle.

Treatment Resistance or Complications

If there is no improvement with topical anti-inflammatories, as well as symptomatic management and gentle vulvar care, intralesional anti-inflammatories should be tried. Patients can apply lidocaine 2% jelly 30 minutes before their appointment to limit the discomfort during injections. If there is no improvement with anti-inflammatory

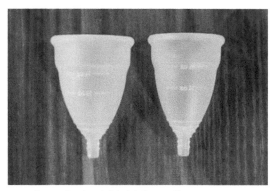

Fig. 3. Silicone menstrual cups in size 1 (*right*) for nulliparous or younger than age 30 years women and size 2 (*left*) for primiparous or multiparous and older than age 30 years women. Inserted into the vagina to collect menstrual fluid.

A   B

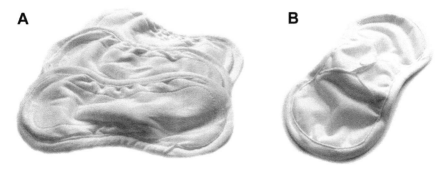

Fig. 4. (*A*, *B*) Reusable cloth pads.

therapy, the diagnosis should always be revisited. Speculum examination with wet mount, as well as skin biopsy, should be performed to rule out any occult dermatoses.

EVALUATION OF OUTCOME AND LONG-TERM RECOMMENDATIONS

Outcome evaluations are from both patient-reported feelings of improvement (or lack thereof), as well as signs of decreased erythema, excoriations, and lichenification on physical examination. Improvement in sleep quality, as well as ability to engage in baseline sexual function, should be assessed. Unlike the inflammatory conditions LP and LS, vulvar pruritus and LSC do not pose a risk of scarring or cancer long-term. However, recurrence of symptoms is common even after a complete remission.

SUMMARY

In summary, vulvar pruritus and LSC are common reasons for presentation to women's health practitioners. The cause of both is often multifactorial and confounded by other inflammatory, neoplastic, infectious, environmental, neuro-pathic, hormonal, and behavioral variables. Treatment must be directed by first ruling out secondary causes of pruritus and then at decreasing inflammation, reducing irri-tants, and providing symptomatic relief to achieve optimal results. With multifaceted care, remission is possible and patients can be reassured that there is little overall health risk from these conditions.

REFERENCES

1. Chen ZQ, Liu XY, Jeffry J, et al. Descending control of itch transmission by the serotonergic system via 5-HT1A-facilitated GRP-GRPR signaling. Neuron 2014; 84(4):821–34.
2. Edwards L, Lynch PJ. Genital pruritus and the eczematous diseases. Genital Dermatology Atlas. 2nd edition. Philadelphia: Lippincott, Williams, & Wilkins; 2011.
3. How to prevent sexually transmitted infections (STIs). FAQ gynecologic problems (FAQ009). ACOG; 2015. Available at: http://www.acog.org/Patients/FAQs/How-to-Prevent-Sexually-Transmitted-Infections-STIs. Accessed December, 2016.
4. Weisshaar E, Mettang T, Tschulena U, et al. Health-related quality of life in haemo-dialysis patients suffering from chronic itch: results from GEHIS (German Epide-miology Haemodialysis Itch Study). Qual Life Res 2016;25(12):3097–106.

5. Vaginal Health. Monistat. Available at: http://www.monistat.com/vaginal-health. Accessed December, 2016.

6. Allergen of the year. ACDS website. Available at: http://www.contactderm.org/i4a/pages/index.cfm?pageid=3467A. Accessed December, 2016.

7. Microscopy, KOH, and pH testing. Vulvovaginal disorders: an algorithm for basic adult diagnosis and treatment. Available at: http://www.vulvovaginaldisorders.com. Accessed December, 2016.

8. Xue F, Li Q, Shang X, et al. Verrucous carcinoma of the vulva: a 20 year retrospective study and literature review. J Low Genit Tract Dis 2016;20(1):114–8.

9. Cribier B, Frouin E, Bodin F, et al. Syringoma: a clinicopathological study of 244 cases. Ann Dermatol Venereol 2016;143(8–9):521–8.

10. Johnston R. Psoriasiform reaction pattern. Weedon's skin pathology essentials. London: Elsevier; 2012.

11. Levine N. The tale of the $220 tube of clobetasol cream. 2015. Available at: http://dermatologytimes.modernmedicine.com/dermatology-times/news/tale-220-tube-clobetasol-cream-2. Accessed December, 2016.

Genital Lichen Sclerosus and its Mimics

Anuja Vyas, MD

KEYWORDS

- Genital lichen sclerosus mimics • Vulvar lichen sclerosus
- Lichen sclerosus similar diagnosis • Vulvar dermatoses

KEY POINTS

- Vulvar dermatoses are common.
- Vulvar dermatoses can be difficult to distinguish from one another; lichen sclerosus alone can be mistaken for myriad disorders.
- Lichen sclerosus can appear similarly to lichen planus, contact dermatitis, Paget disease, and others.
- Biopsies are important but can be misleading.
- Therapies should be tailored accordingly.
- Close relationships between gynecologists, dermatologists, and pathologists create the ideal multidisciplinary team to care for women with any of the above conditions.

INTRODUCTION

Lichen sclerosus is a benign but chronic and often progressive dermatologic condition. In most cases, lichen sclerosus occurs in the anogenital region (85%–98% reported in the literature) but can develop on any skin surface.[1,2] Extragenital lichen sclerosus is not as prevalent and will not be discussed here, as it is not the primary focus of this article.

Vulvar lichen sclerosus (VLS) is characterized by marked inflammation, epithelial thinning, and distinct dermal alterations often accompanied by varying degrees of pruritus and pain.

A variety of disorders may be confused with VLS, as they can share several common features. This article discusses diagnosis, workup, and management of VLS with specific attention on distinguishing it from other dermatologic mimics.

CLINICAL MANIFESTATIONS

Careful examination of the vulvar skin in women with VLS will show characteristic findings along with architectural changes. Classic VLS can be identified by white,

Disclosure Statement: No disclosures.
Department of Obstetrics and Gynecology, Baylor College of Medicine, 3771 Elmora Street, Houston, TX 77005, USA
E-mail addresses: avyas@bcm.edu; sanghvi.anuja@gmail.com

atrophic-appearing papules that may coalesce into plaques to create a thin wrinkled appearance to the skin. Early in the disease course, vulvar architecture tends to remain intact. However, as the disease progresses, the distinction between the labia majora and minora is lost to varying degrees, and the clitoris can become buried under a fused prepuce. In more severe, uncontrolled, or end-stage VLS, the vulva appears pale, can be completely fused in the midline (because of labia minora agglutination) with only a pinhole vaginal orifice. Uncontrolled VLS will also exhibit excoriations from chronic scratching, edema from inflammation, purpural lesions, and ecchymoses given the fragility of the affected skin.

VLS lesions most frequently affect the labia minora. Fordyce spots, which represent normal sebaceous glands, disappear along the inner labia minora. Some women manifest whitening that extends over the perineum and around the anus in what is termed a *keyhole* fashion. Fissuring is common at the posterior vestibular fourchette, interlabial folds, around the clitoris, and in the perianal region. Extension into the genitocrural folds and buttocks is rare. True vaginal involvement of lichen sclerosus is uncommon.[3]

Although some women are asymptomatic, vulvar itching continues to be the hallmark symptom of the disease. Soreness and irritation place at a close second. Often itching can be intense to the point of creating sleep interference. Pruritus ani, pain with defecation, anal fissures, and rectal bleeding are common with perianal involvement. With advanced disease—specifically when labia minora fusion over urethral meatus has occurred—women can have dysuria and difficulty voiding.

Sexual dysfunction is common in women with VLS. Chronic posterior vestibular fissures and concurrent scarring lead to decreased tissue pliability. The posterior vestibule is the anatomic site on the vagina that receives the most friction and trauma during the act of vaginal penetration. Lack of pliability in this region compounded with repeated unwanted friction eventually increases nerve sensitivity to this vaginal entryway and pain to the point of sexual aversion. Both generalized and localized secondary vulvodynia can result from VLS disease–related neuromuscular dysfunction. Other architectural changes such as a narrowed vaginal introitus along with atrophic changes from estrogen deficiency can additionally result in significant dyspareunia. Some women complain of decreased sexual sensation and orgasm because of fusion of the clitoral hood over the clitoris. The negative impact on overall quality of life cannot be underestimated (**Figs. 1** and **2** and **Table 1**).[4]

DIAGNOSIS

A 4-mm punch biopsy typically provides sufficient tissue to confirm the diagnosis of VLS. Clinical and pathologic correlation in conjunction with a dermatopathologist is ideal. Typical histologic findings include a thinned epidermis with areas of hyperkeratosis and acanthosis.[5] The upper dermis will exhibit homogenization of collagen with underlying lymphocytic infiltration.

Characteristic histologic findings vary dramatically in VLS. Often, pathology differs on the clinical stage of VLS at the time of biopsy. For example, in early VLS, the findings can be subtle and nonspecific. In later or older stages of disease, lymphocytic infiltration may be absent, but dermal sclerosis will be readily apparent. This happens often when VLS has been present for extended periods (eg, since childhood). Histology can also vary if the biopsy misses the area of active disease or in cases of recent topical corticosteroid treatment.[6]

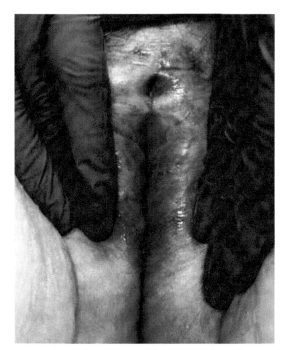

Fig. 1. Lichen sclerosus with agglutination of labia in midline. (*Courtesy of* A. Vyas, MD, Houston, TX.)

A small subset of patients exhibit mainly hypertrophic VLS. Whereas most biopsy results in women with VLS show atrophy and epidermal thinning, women with the hypertrophic variant have marked epidermal thickening (acanthosis) instead. In fact, it is this finding that primarily led to current terminology change from *lichen sclerosus et atrophicus* to the more straightforward and inclusive *vulvar lichen sclerosus*. Hyperkeratotic VLS lesions can require more aggressive therapy. Treatment of VLS is discussed separately.

Given the above findings, the diagnosis of VLS will often be based solely on the presence of characteristic clinical manifestations. Clinical judgment should guide diagnosis and management of VLS when biopsy results are not specific. However, biopsies should be reperformed in cases of treatment failure, to confirm or re-evaluate the VLS diagnosis, and to rule out malignancy. Of note, prepubertal children do not need biopsy confirmation of VLS, as their clinical findings tend to be entirely classic.

There is no laboratory test or value that is specific to the diagnosis of VLS. However, it is well known that autoimmune disorders are more common among patients with VLS.[7,8] Laboratory assessments and additional diagnostic studies should look for specific autoimmune disorders when the patient reports clinical signs or symptoms suggestive of them. For example, thyroid disease is common among women with VLS.[9] If a patient has a positive review of systems that may indicate thyroid disorder, the practice should be to order laboratory tests looking for this condition. Investigative studies such as genital cultures or microscopic wet mount should be performed if there are signs of vulvar or vaginal infection. Attendant infections are common in women with VLS.[10]

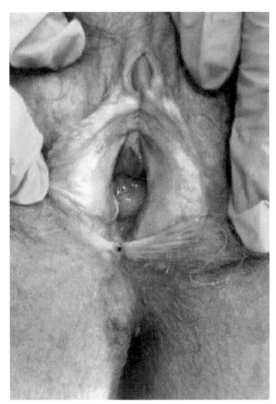

Fig. 2. Lichen sclerosus with posterior vestibular fissuring. (*Courtesy of* A. Vyas, MD, Houston, TX.)

Table 1
Vulvar lichen sclerosus signs and symptoms

Signs	Symptoms
Thin, white, wrinkled vulvar skin that can extend in "keyhole" fashion over perianal area	Pruritus with soreness and irritation
White atrophic papules and/or plaques	Sexual dysfunction—loss of sensation, dyspareunia
Loss of distinction between labia majora and minora	Dysuria and difficulty voiding
Fused clitoral prepuce—clitoris will appear buried	Vulvodynia—chronic or provoked burning sensation
Complete agglutination of labia minora in midline with pallor of surrounding skin	
Excoriations and fissures	
Edema	
Ecchymoses, purpural lesions	

MANAGEMENT

Goals of therapy should be 2-fold:

1. To resolve VLS symptoms of itching and vulvar and vaginal pain
2. To reduce signs of disease including hyperkeratosis, fissuring, and ecchymoses

In adults, scarring and loss of architecture persist despite therapy. In children however, architectural changes such as labial adhesions may actually improve.

Initial management, like with other conditions, involves patient education. Given the current level of access to unfiltered information via internet resources, women often worry excessively regarding disease implications. Every effort should be made to discuss the patient's individual situation. Clinical photography and use of a handheld mirror for the patient to visualize their anatomy with the help of a trained practitioner can be very beneficial. It is important to discuss the chronic nature of VLS with periods of flares—recurrences and remissions of signs and symptoms. Reassurance regarding how manageable the disorder is in most cases will go a long way in mitigating patient distress. Good vulvar hygiene methods should be discussed. The associated risk of malignancy (ie, vulvar squamous cell carcinoma) and need for clinical follow-up every 6 months to yearly should be mentioned. Patients should also be educated on vulvar self-awareness and the need to return more frequently to their physician's office for nonhealing sores, bleeding, or recalcitrant itching despite therapy.

Medical therapy should be concurrently initiated with patient education. Topical corticosteroids, specifically ones from the superpotent group and in ointment form, are the mainstay of therapy. Clobetasol propionate 0.05% has long been the standard of care for treatment of VLS. Clobetasol is a class I, superpotent corticosteroid. Other equivalent and effective steroids in the same class include betamethasone dipropionate 0.05% and halobetasol 0.05% in ointment form. Topical steroids can be highly effective and can even inhibit progression of disease.[11–16] Many women find vulvar creams irritating. This is possibly because they can be excessively drying because of the alcohol bases they are regularly prepared in.

Before recommending less potent topical corticosteroids as first-line medical therapy for VLS, more studies need to be performed documenting similar efficacy to the superpotent options. Thick hypertrophic plaques may need intralesional steroid injections (eg, triamcinolone) or retinoids, as topical corticosteroid therapies may not adequately penetrate these areas. Treatment regimens vary and should be tailored to the individual's disease appearance.

In general, the superpotent steroid ointment should be applied to the affected areas (shown to the patient with a mirror to ensure appropriate administration) in a small, less than pea-sized amount (approximately 1 fingertip unit) 2 times per day for 6 to 12 weeks. The patient should liberally apply a topical moisturizer like clear petroleum jelly afterward—both to seal in moisture and to propagate the steroid's effect as the skin becomes more hydrated over time. Follow-up in the doctor's office is required after this initial therapeutic phase to ensure appropriate application technique by the patient, progress of symptom relief, and hopefully remission of some vulvar skin changes. The topical steroid can then be tapered down to once daily use over 2 to 4 weeks with further backing down of product use to every other day, then 2 to 3 times per week for long-term maintenance. Alternatively, the patient can initiate use of a milder potency topical corticosteroid daily (eg, triamcinolone acetonide 0.1%, class IV) instead of tapering the frequency of a class I product once disease has been adequately controlled. This method may be useful for those women who have difficulty remembering to apply a medication to their genitalia unless it is a daily habit. Because the ideal regimen is not known, experienced providers typically have their own methods for treating, tapering, and maintaining. Maintenance therapy is indicated to prevent symptom recurrence and decrease incidence of vulvar intraepithelial neoplasia and vulvar cancer.[17] With flares, the patient should be instructed to increase the frequency of topical steroid application, not the amount. Written instructions should be used routinely, as patients are often overwhelmed with the volume of information received during consultation visits.

Adverse effects from overuse of potent topical steroids can occur. This overuse is another reason patients need to be educated on the importance of close clinical follow-up and medication compliance. The modified mucous membranes of the labia and clitoris are relatively resistant to steroid-related side effects, but hair-bearing skin of the labia majora, perianal skin, and groin fold creases are prone to steroid-induced atrophy. Atrophic changes and contact dermatitis from steroid overuse in these areas are easily identifiable during monitoring. As a universal rule, it is always best to aim for the lowest frequency and potency of steroid application that will keep symptoms and examination findings under good control. Tailoring therapy to the individual patient is of utmost importance.

After education on disease chronicity and management, it is best not to ignore the loss of intimacy, associated feelings of guilt, and sexual dysfunction components of VLS. Women with significant menopausal-related vulvovaginal atrophy can and should be prescribed an appropriate hormone regimen. Systemic menopause therapy should be addressed as needed. Therapeutic options are broad and should be customized to the patient and physician's individualized preferences. Information on lubricants for sexual pleasure should be given to women regardless of their preference on hormone therapy. Patients may also require a referral to a sexual counselor. Acknowledging the impact of VLS on a woman's emotional well-being is a critically important piece of the doctor-patient relationship. Information regarding local and national patient support groups should also be provided to the patient.

Second-line therapies are not often needed given the high therapeutic efficacy of local corticosteroid therapy. If other causes of treatment failure are ruled out (eg, infection, alternate diagnosis, improper application, poor tolerability of steroid), calcineurin inhibitors can be used. Calcineurin inhibitors like tacrolimus and pimecrolimus may not be as effective as topical superpotent steroid therapy, are more expensive, and are less well tolerated on the vulvar skin. Long-term safety regarding topical use is still being questioned.[18]

Other therapies have been used for management of VLS; however, lack of expansive efficacy data, lack of convenience, and potential for associated adverse effects have limited their use. These options include oral acitretin, topical hormone therapies, ultraviolet phototherapy, photodynamic therapy, carbon dioxide laser, and surgery involving use of fat-derived stem cells and platelet-rich plasma.[19] Oral corticosteroids are not used for routine management of VLS given the significant risk for systemic side effects. In cases of recalcitrant VLS, oral steroid tapers with subsequent maintenance of symptoms using an immune modulator like methotrexate can be clinically beneficial.[20,21]

DIFFERENTIAL DIAGNOSES

Recognizing the differences between common vulvar disorders is important for any gynecologist but especially so for the provider who wishes to be known as a vulvologist. A skilled clinician should be able to distinguish the variety of other disorders that can be confused with VLS. Although a diagnostic biopsy can be very useful, they can be relatively nonspecific as mentioned above. This section outlines vulvar skin conditions that mimic VLS and ways to distinguish between them.

Lichen Planus

There are many subtypes of lichen planus, any of which can affect the vulva. The most common form seen in the genital area is erosive genital lichen planus (ELP) (**Fig. 3**).[22] ELP and VLS share several common features (**Fig. 4**). They may even occur together on the vulva. Both are postulated to occur from an autoimmune disturbance. Symptoms of intense pruritus, irritation, burning, and pain are common. Loss of vulvar architecture happens as well. ELP tends to be more difficult to control with relapses and remittances as the norm. ELP also usually involves the vagina in the form of erythematous and friable lesions, inflammatory vaginal discharge, or synechiae, which can be extensive to the point of complete obliteration. Whereas most cases of VLS are adequately controlled with return to baseline function, ELP can be more devastating both sexually and physically.[23] A punch biopsy can be helpful to distinguish between these disorders, but histologic findings may be similar. Clinical management should guide management in these cases. Treatment involves topical and intravaginal steroids with systemic immune-modulating therapies for intractable cases.

Lichen Simplex Chronicus

Lichen simplex chronicus is not considered a primary skin disorder. It is commonly noted in adult forms of atopic dermatitis.[24] The same itch-scratch cycle as occurs

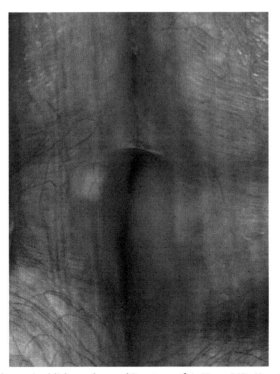

Fig. 3. Erosive vulvovaginal lichen planus. (*Courtesy of* A. Vyas, MD, Houston, TX.)

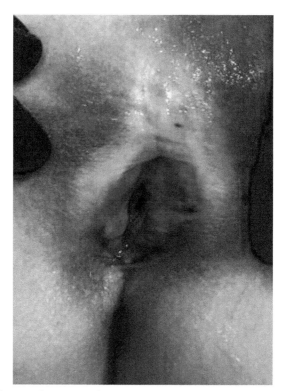

Fig. 4. Lichen sclerosus. (*Courtesy of* A. Vyas, MD, Houston, TX.)

in atopic dermatitis leads to vigorous scratching and rubbing. Some patients state they will rub so as not to scratch where others have resorted to using scrubbing brushes to gain relief from the itch sensation. Patients often complain that their symptoms are worse at night. Psychological factors such as depression or obsessive compulsive disorder may contribute to lichen simplex chronicus.[25] With vulvar lichen simplex chronicus, women typically complain of intense pruritus in the groin area. On physical examination, the vulvar skin, particularly the hair- bearing labia and groin, will exhibit lichenified plaques of thickened skin and excoriations from excessive scratching. Excoriations can even result in ulcers. Affected vulvar skin can appear edematous and leathery in appearance from chronic inflammation (**Fig. 5**). In contrast to VLS, vulvar anatomy and architecture in vulvar lichen simplex chronicus will be preserved, which is an important feature in making the diagnosis.

Vulvar lichen simplex chronicus does not involve the vagina. A patient may, however, have an active genital infection at the time of presentation. A thorough history may reveal the onset of vulvar itching in conjunction with an infection. Once the infection is treated, however, vaginal symptoms will resolve. In vulvar lichen simplex chronicus, external itching and scratching will continue despite the absence of an active vaginal infection.

Lichen simplex chronicus is diagnosed based on clinical findings with rare need for biopsy. Histologic specimens show elongation, widening, and irregular thickening of rete ridges (acanthosis), hyperkeratosis, parakeratosis, and middermal inflammatory infiltrate. Breaking the cycle of scratching is the central goal of treatment. Commonly used therapies include topical and intralesional corticosteroids. Generally, steroids are

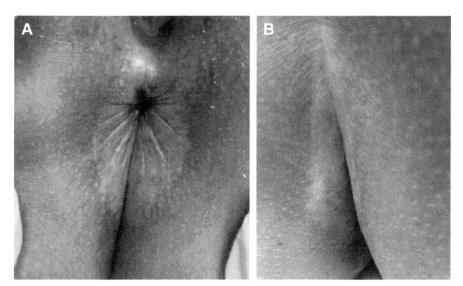

Fig. 5. (*A, B*) Perianal lichen simplex chronicus. (*Courtesy of* A. Vyas, MD, Houston, TX.)

tapered off but maintenance may be required for months. Long-term maintenance is not required, as this disease entity does not progress to squamous cell dysplasia.

Endogenous and Exogenous Dermatitis

Vulvar dermatitis can be indistinguishable from early VLS. Clinical findings vary and can range from erythema and scaling to fissuring and thick lichenified tissue. Whereas with VLS the labia minora are most commonly affected, in pure vulvar dermatitis, the labia majora are more commonly involved. The cause is typically multifactorial. Endogenous disorders like atopic dermatitis and exogenous factors like contact or allergic irritants contribute to findings.

It is interesting that vulvar tissue seems to function less efficiently as a barrier when compared with other body regions. Vulvar skin tends to be particularly susceptible to irritants and allergens.[26] Therefore, steroid overuse and calcineurin inhibitors are poorly tolerated and cause noticeable skin changes in the sensitive vulvar tissue.

Any suspicion of neoplasia should warrant a biopsy. In most cases, however, biopsy is unnecessary to make the diagnosis of contact, irritant-based, or atopic dermatitis. For contact dermatitis, removal of the offending agent will often suffice with or without a short course of a mild potency steroid ointment application. In cases of atopy, intermittent mild potency steroid application with flares is the mainstay of therapy (**Fig. 6**).

Estrogen Deficiency

Of striking importance is just how many board-certified gynecologists do not recognize the differences between normal age-related vulvar changes and VLS. In our practice, as part of tertiary care referral center, women have been told repeatedly that their clinical symptoms and physical examination findings are related to hypoestrogenism. Only if the skin disease has advanced to the point of complete loss of labial and clitoral architecture or a vulvar biopsy was done will a patient be told they have VLS.

In the estrogen-depleted state, vulvar tissues lose elasticity and fat. This loss is particularly noticeable in the labia majora. The clitoris may appear shrunken, but

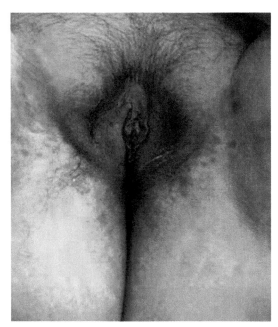

Fig. 6. Vulvar contact dermatitis. (*Courtesy of* A. Vyas, MD, Houston, TX.)

the prepuce will not be fused over. The labia minora may lose some of their natural pink color and appear pale, but fusion in the midline or outward to create no demarcation between the labia will not occur solely because of menopausal state. Even if fusion does occur, it will be mild and should resolve within 2 weeks of estrogen therapy.

Menopause often induces a change in coloration around vestibular gland and urethral openings. The vaginal mucosa surrounding the Bartholin glands will appear red as will the mucosa immediately surrounding the urethral meatus. The vagina itself will lose typical ruggae and may exhibit minimal or a mild yellow exudate from epithelial cell sloughing. The vaginal pH will invariably be increased to greater than 4.5 as estrogen-dependent lactobacilli are diminished. Symptomatically, patients may complain of frequent urinary tract or genital infections, a raw or burning sensation with vaginal intercourse, and possibly an itching sensation. VLS and hypoestrogenism will likely be coincident; however, many if not most of the uncomfortable symptoms and signs of estrogen deficiency will resolve with the addback of vaginal or topical estrogen. Hormone therapy alone will not improve VLS. An anti-inflammatory agent (most often a superpotent steroid) will be needed to control symptoms. Physical examination findings in VLS, especially scarring, will not return to normal state.

Vitiligo

Vitiligo lesions can appear anywhere on the body but do have a predilection for the genital area, face, orifices, and hands. Because vitiligo in the vulvar area produces whitening, it can be confused with VLS. The depigmented white changes of vitiligo, however, will lack the classic clinical signs of inflammation that go along with VLS unless they coexist in the same patient. Case reports of co-occurrence are reported in the literature. The commonality may lie in their autoimmunogenicity.[27–29]

In contrast to VLS, which has a predilection for hypoestrogenic states, vitiligo lesions can appear at any age. In addition, a careful history may uncover that onset of vitiligo lesions was associated with some degree of skin trauma (such as severe sunburn), recent pregnancy, or emotional stress. This association of onset in proximity to recent trauma has been dubbed the *Koebner phenomenon*.

The diagnosis of vitiligo is mostly straightforward—discrete, well-demarcated white macules on various body parts without inflammatory changes. The diagnosis can be further facilitated by use of a Wood ultraviolet lamp. Under ultraviolet A light, depigmented areas will emit a bright blue-white fluorescence. Skin biopsies are not routinely needed, but hypopigmented or depigmented lesions of unclear etiology should be further evaluated. Autoimmune thyroid disease is frequently associated with vitiligo. The current consensus is to screen for thyroid function in all patients with vitiligo.[30] Therapies to treat vitiligo are manifold.[31] Mid to super high-potency topical steroids are used as first-line therapy. Calcineurin inhibitors, phototherapy, replenishment of vitamins D, E, C, B12, folic acid, and herbal supplements are often used to help with repigmentation or halt disease progression. Surgery remains a viable option for patients with localized disease unresponsive to conventional therapies.

Candidiasis

Because vulvovaginal candidiasis is characterized by chronic vulvar itching and vulvar burning and is the more common diagnosis in a general gynecologic population, women may be treated repetitively for candida before making the diagnosis of VLS. Women do not always have the classic white, curdlike vaginal discharge. For example, *Candida glabrata* may exhibit little or mild watery discharge. On physical examination, vulvar and vaginal erythema with edema may be sufficiently present to slightly distort vulvar anatomy, making it even harder to distinguish VLS from candidiasis.

Clinically useful tools include the in-office wet mount and examination of vaginal pH. Unfortunately, many recently trained gynecologists lack knowledge of these diagnostic commodities. Candida species typically create a low vaginal pH; however, if not treated with estrogen, women with VLS will have a high vaginal pH level from hypoestrogenism. Candida will create a vaginal discharge, whereas VLS patients will have little to no moisture coating the vaginal walls. Treatment of uncomplicated vulvovaginal candidiasis is with topical or oral imidazoles. Both VLS and candida can coexist, and yeast infections can cause flares of VLS symptoms. If clinical suspicion for VLS remains after treatment of candidiasis, a vulvar biopsy can help confirm the diagnosis.

Psoriasis

Psoriasis is a common chronic skin disorder with a variety of clinical forms. It is typical to find well-demarcated erythematous plaques often with a silvery scale on various body parts. The scales erupt most often on the scalp, extensor elbows, knees, and back. When the vulva is involved, psoriasis tends to affect the hair-bearing labia and intertriginous groin areas (**Fig. 7**). Because this presentation can be different or reverse of that found in the usual psoriatic presentation on extensor surfaces, it is called *inverse psoriasis*. Inverse psoriasis may not have any clinical symptoms (pruritus and sexual dysfunction may be absent), whereas uncontrolled VLS will invariably create itching and sexual dysfunction. Inverse psoriasis can affect any age group and does not have a predilection for hypoestrogenic states.

Typical clinical findings result from hyperproliferation and hyperplasia of the epidermis, neutrophilic infiltrates with our without microabscesses, plasma cell infiltrates, and vascular changes. These findings are in contrast to the histologic findings

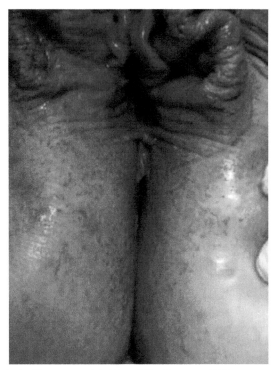

Fig. 7. Vulvar psoriasis. (*Courtesy of* A. Vyas, MD, Houston, TX.)

of VLS—a thinned epidermis with subepidermal homogenization and collagenation with variable numbers of plasma cell infiltrates.[32,33]

Much more is known about the pathophysiology of psoriasis than that of VLS, leading to numerous therapies.[34] The mainstays, however, continue to be topical steroids, calcineurin inhibitors, and emollients. Phototherapy and a variety of systemic immune-modifying agents are also used. In women with moderate-to-severe vulvar psoriasis, it is best to coordinate care between the gynecologist and a dermatologist.

Paget Disease

The differential diagnosis of VLS should include vulvar Paget disease. Although most often associated with the breast, Paget disease can affect extramammary tissues, specifically the bone and vulva. Vulvar Paget disease has an eczematous appearance and will be well demarcated with slightly raised edges in a red background. Paget disease of the vulva primarily afflicts white women in their later menopausal years (60s and 70s). As in VLS, pruritus is the most common symptom. Secondary symptoms include discharge from the lesions, burning, and pain. Paget disease is generally multifocal with occurrence anywhere on the vulva, mons, perineum, and inner thighs but less so surrounding the clitoris. VLS typically spares the mons and inner thighs but has a predilection for the clitoris and perineum. Paget disease also has a much higher inherent association with vulvar cancer (namely, adenocarcinoma) than VLS—up to 17% quoted in the literature. Thankfully, it only accounts for less than 1% of all vulvar malignancies.[35]

Table 2
Features of vulvar dermatoses

Vulvar Diagnosis	Clinical Findings	Disease Course	Etiology	Histologic Findings	Treatment
Lichen sclerosus	Vulvar itching, soreness, irritation, fissures, dysuria, dyspareunia; architectural disruption and scarring	Chronic, may be progressive if not treated	Unknown, immune dysfunction, genetic, infectious or trauma	Thin epidermis, hyperkeratosis, loss of rete pegs, basal cell degeneration, a homogenized layer of collagen in the upper dermis with a band of lymphocytes below	Topical corticosteroids, calcineurin inhibitors, retinoids, immune modulators, limited data on laser therapy
Estrogen deficiency	Vaginal dryness, burning, irritation; decreased lubrication; dyspareunia; postcoital bleeding; fissures; discharge; urinary symptoms	Progressive if not treated	Extremes of age, medically or surgically induced leading to decreased ovarian production of sex hormones	Thin vaginal epithelium with increased parabasal cells and decreased superficial and intermediate epithelial cells	Hormone supplementation, vaginal lubricants, moisturizers
Yeast dermatitis	Pruritus, burning, soreness, irritation, dysuria; vulvar edema, excoriations, fissures, ± vaginal discharge	Sporadic or recurrent	Candida or other species (eg, saccharomyces)	Vaginal epithelial smear shows budding yeast, pseudohyphae, hyphae after administration of 10% potassium hydroxide	Topical or oral azoles, vaginal boric acid, gentian violet, nystatin, flucytosine, amphotericin, and echinocandins
Lichen planus	Pruritus, burning, pain, soreness, dysuria, dyspareunia; bright, erythematous erosions with white striae (Wickham striae), architectural disruption and scarring, vaginal stenosis and copious discharge	Chronic, relapsing and remitting	Unknown; autoimmune postulated (T-cell-mediated attack against basal keratinocytes)	Biopsy shows irregular epidermal acanthosis and scattered apoptotic keratinocytes, vacuolar change of epidermal basal cell layer, bandlike lymphocytic dermal infiltrate in upper dermis; various degrees of plasma cell infiltration in mucosal biopsies	Topical corticosteroids, calcineurin inhibitors, topical or systemic immune-modifying agents

(continued on next page)

Table 2
(continued)

Vulvar Diagnosis	Clinical Findings	Disease Course	Etiology	Histologic Findings	Treatment
Lichen simplex chronicus	Intense pruritus (marked at night), bleeding from excoriations; lichenified plaques	Acute, subacute, chronic	Itch-scratch cycle initiated by offending agent or neuropathic, atopic	Biopsy shows hyperkeratosis, prominent granular cell layer, elongation and irregular thickening of epidermal rete, mild spongiotic changes, perivascular inflammation (histiocytes, lymphocytes, eosinophils) in superficial dermis	Topical corticosteroids, if severe then oral pulse dosed or intramuscular corticosteroids can be indicated
Vitiligo	Asymptomatic depigmented macules and patches that lack clinical signs of inflammation (chalk white or milky in color)	Unpredictable (acute skin alteration that remains stable or is chronic and progressively affects more surface area)	Unknown; autoimmune and/or oxidative stress (Koebner phenomenon) postulated (leading to destruction of melanocytes)	Biopsy shows decreased to no melanocytes, degenerative changes in nerves and sweat glands, increased Langerhans cells	Topical corticosteroids, phototherapy, autologous transplant of healthy melanocytes in depigmented skin
Contact dermatitis	Pruritus (intense and nocturnal), burning, stinging, rawness with exacerbations caused by heat, sweat, stress, menstruation; vulvar erythema, scaling, fissures, excoriations, exaggerated and swollen labial folds, sparse pubic hair, postinflammatory pigmentary changes, secondary infection	Acute, subacute	Allergens or irritant based	Biopsy shows epidermal edema (spongiosis) and dermal lymphocytic infiltrate and occasional eosinophils	Removal of inciting agent, mid- to high-potency topical corticosteroids, oral antipruritic agents, systemic steroids for refractory disease

	Clinical features	Course	Etiology	Biopsy	Treatment
Psoriasis	Asymptomatic, sometimes pruritic; erythematous plaques with sharply defined margins and silvery scale	Unpredictable but generally chronic	Genetic, autoimmune, Koebner phenomenon, multifactorial	Biopsy shows parakeratosis, acanthosis with downward elongation of rete ridges resembling a comb, neutrophilic microabscesses in parakeratotic scales, mixed dermal infiltrate (lymphocytes, macrophages, neutrophils)	Topical corticosteroids, emollients, systemic immune-modifying agents, phototherapy
Paget disease	Pruritus; eczematoid lesions, well-demarcated with slightly raised edges in a red background, small pale islands	Subacute with latency 6–8 mo before diagnosis on average	Genetic, malignant transformation of epidermal keratinocytes	Biopsy shows large, atypical cells spread out in epidermis, cells appear clear with mucin and sometimes melanin, large nucleus	Laser, ultrasonic aspirator therapy, surgical excision, topical imiquimod
Mucus membrane pemphigoid	Pain, pruritus; tense blisters and erosions, healed lesions will scar, desquamative vaginitis	Acute and self limited, more often chronic, progressive with frequent exacerbations and remissions	Autoimmune (circulating autoantibodies against basement membrane proteins), adverse medication effect (reaction to penicillamine)	Biopsy of lesion shows spongiosis and subepidermal blisters with numerous eosinophils, variable dermal cell infiltrate of lymphocytes, eosinophils and neutrophils Perilesional biopsy shows linear IgG, IgA, and/or C3 staining along basement membrane	Topical, systemic steroids, immune suppressive agents

Histologically, Paget cells located within epidermal tissue are pathognomonic for the disease. Paget cells have a classic vacuolated appearance with pale/clear cytoplasm and prominent nucleoli. Younger women or those concerned about cosmesis may be candidates for alternative surgical-sparing procedures like laser, ultrasonic aspirators, or pharmacologic therapy. This management must be heavily weighed against the malignant potential of Paget disease. Excisional procedures are preferred including vulvarwide local excision, skinning, or simple vulvectomy depending on extent of lesions.

Mucous Membrane Pemphigoid

Mucous membrane pemphigoid (MMP) is uncommon. It represents a heterogeneous group of chronic subepithelial blistering disorders that affect mucosal surfaces. Symptoms are relapsing and remitting mucosal inflammation and erosions with frequent scarring.

The diagnosis should be considered if there is marked labial adhesion or nonresponsiveness to topical steroids. Biopsy distinguishes between VLS and pemphigoid. If one is considering MMP as a potential diagnosis, ideally 2 specimens should be obtained—a lesional skin biopsy from the edge of an intact blister or other inflamed tissue for routine pathology and staining (hematoxylin and eosin) and a perilesional tissue biopsy for direct immunofluorescence. The tissue specimen for direct immunofluorescence should not be placed in formalin but instead in a transport medium compatible for immunofluorescence studies. In 80% to 90% of MMP cases, linear IgG, IgA, or C3 staining along the basement membrane zone is detected.[36,37] In addition, serum samples in patients with MMP should be sent for indirect immunofluorescence and enzyme-linked immunosorbent assay testing to detect circulating basement membrane zone antibodies.[36] Treatment is with local topical steroids or systemic immune-modulating therapies such as oral steroids or glucocorticoid-sparing agents. Refractory disease may necessitate more aggressive therapy like intravenous immune globulin therapy.

MMP will more often be confused with lichen planus than with VLS, as both MMP and lichen planus more frequently involve the mucus membranes of the oral and genital cavity, are chronically relapsing and remitting, and can cause a desquamative vaginal discharge.

SUMMARY

Vulvar dermatoses are exceedingly common and can impersonate one another. Lichen sclerosus alone can be mistaken for myriad disorders. Close relationships between gynecologists, dermatologists, and pathologists create the ideal multidisciplinary team to care for women with any of the above conditions (**Table 2**).

REFERENCES

1. Ridley CM, Neill SM, Lewis FM. Ridley's the vulva. 3rd edition. Chichester (United Kingdom): Wiley-Blackwell; 2009. xi, 280 p.
2. Thomas RH, Ridley CM, McGibbon DH, et al. Anogenital lichen sclerosus in women. J R Soc Med 1996;89:694–8.
3. Funaro D. Lichen sclerosus: a review and practical approach. Dermatol Ther 2004;17:28–37.
4. Haefner HK, Aldrich NZ, Dalton VK, et al. The impact of vulvar lichen sclerosus on sexual dysfunction. J Womens Health (Larchmt) 2014;23:765–70.

5. Regauer S, Liegl B, Reich O. Early vulvar lichen sclerosus: a histopathological challenge. Histopathology 2005;47:340–7.
6. Greene L. Vulvar inflammatory dermatoses for the nondermatopathologist: an approach for the practising surgical pathologist. Diagn Histopathology 2010; 16:487–94.
7. Karadag AS, Kavala M, Ozlu E, et al. The co-occurrence of lichen sclerosus et atrophicus and celiac disease. Indian Dermatol Online J 2014;5:S106–8.
8. Jacobs L, Gilliam A, Khavari N, et al. Association between lichen sclerosus and celiac disease: a report of three pediatric cases. Pediatr Dermatol 2014;31: e128–31.
9. Birenbaum DL, Young RC. High prevalence of thyroid disease in patients with lichen sclerosus. J Reprod Med 2007;52:28–30.
10. Fistarol SK, Itin PH. Diagnosis and treatment of lichen sclerosus: an update. Am J Clin Dermatol 2013;14:27–47.
11. Neill SM, Lewis FM, Tatnall FM, et al, British Association of Dermatologists. British Association of Dermatologists' guidelines for the management of lichen sclerosus 2010. Br J Dermatol 2010;163:672–82.
12. Zellis S, Pincus SH. Treatment of vulvar dermatoses. Semin Dermatol 1996;15: 71–6.
13. Bracco GL, Carli P, Sonni L, et al. Clinical and histologic effects of topical treatments of vulval lichen sclerosus. A critical evaluation. J Reprod Med 1993;38: 37–40.
14. Chi CC, Kirtschig G, Baldo M, et al. Topical interventions for genital lichen sclerosus. Cochrane Database Syst Rev 2011;(12):CD008240.
15. Lorenz B, Kaufman RH, Kutzner SK. Lichen sclerosus. Therapy with clobetasol propionate. J Reprod Med 1998;43:790–4.
16. Goldstein AT, Creasey A, Pfau R, et al. A double-blind, randomized controlled trial of clobetasol versus pimecrolimus in patients with vulvar lichen sclerosus. J Am Acad Dermatol 2011;64:e99–104.
17. Lee A, Bradford J, Fischer G. Long-term management of adult vulvar lichen sclerosus: a prospective cohort study of 507 women. JAMA Dermatol 2015;151: 1061–7.
18. Funaro D, Lovett A, Leroux N, et al. A double-blind, randomized prospective study evaluating topical clobetasol propionate 0.05% versus topical tacrolimus 0.1% in patients with vulvar lichen sclerosus. J Am Acad Dermatol 2014;71: 84–91.
19. Goldstein AT, King M, Runels C, et al. Intradermal injection of autologous platelet-rich plasma for the treatment of vulvar lichen sclerosus. J Am Acad Dermatol 2017;76:158–60.
20. Nayeemuddin F, Yates VM. Lichen sclerosus et atrophicus responding to methotrexate. Clin Exp Dermatol 2008;33:651–2.
21. Kreuter A, Tigges C, Gaifullina R, et al. Pulsed high-dose corticosteroids combined with low-dose methotrexate treatment in patients with refractory generalized extragenital lichen sclerosus. Arch Dermatol 2009;145:1303–8.
22. Simpson RC, Thomas KS, Leighton P, et al. Diagnostic criteria for erosive lichen planus affecting the vulva: an international electronic-Delphi consensus exercise. Br J Dermatol 2013;169:337–43.
23. Lotery HE, Galask RP. Erosive lichen planus of the vulva and vagina. Obstet Gynecol 2003;101:1121–5.
24. Stewart KM. Clinical care of vulvar pruritus, with emphasis on one common cause, lichen simplex chronicus. Dermatol Clin 2010;28:669–80.

25. Konuk N, Koca R, Atik L, et al. Psychopathology, depression and dissociative experiences in patients with lichen simplex chronicus. Gen Hosp Psychiatry 2007; 29:232–5.
26. Elsner P, Wilhelm D, Maibach HI. Multiple parameter assessment of vulvar irritant contact dermatitis. Contact Dermatitis 1990;23:20–6.
27. Weisberg EL, Le LQ, Cohen JB. A case of simultaneously occurring lichen sclerosus and segmental vitiligo: connecting the underlying autoimmune pathogenesis. Int J Dermatol 2008;47:1053–5.
28. Kwon IH, Kye H, Seo SH, et al. Synchronous onset of symmetrically associated extragenital lichen sclerosus and vitiligo on both breasts and the vulva. Ann Dermatol 2015;27:456–7.
29. Cooper SM, Ali I, Baldo M, et al. The association of lichen sclerosus and erosive lichen planus of the vulva with autoimmune disease: a case-control study. Arch Dermatol 2008;144:1432–5.
30. Vrijman C, Kroon MW, Limpens J, et al. The prevalence of thyroid disease in patients with vitiligo: a systematic review. Br J Dermatol 2012;167:1224–35.
31. Whitton M, Pinart M, Batchelor JM, et al. Evidence-based management of vitiligo: summary of a Cochrane systematic review. Br J Dermatol 2016;174:962–9.
32. Iizuka H, Ishida-Yamamoto A, Honda H. Epidermal remodelling in psoriasis. Br J Dermatol 1996;135:433–8.
33. Iizuka H, Takahashi H, Ishida-Yamamoto A. Psoriatic architecture constructed by epidermal remodeling. J Dermatol Sci 2004;35:93–9.
34. Menter A, Griffiths CE. Current and future management of psoriasis. Lancet 2007; 370:272–84.
35. Parker LP, Parker JR, Bodurka-Bevers D, et al. Paget's disease of the vulva: pathology, pattern of involvement, and prognosis. Gynecol Oncol 2000;77:183–9.
36. Schmidt E, della Torre R, Borradori L. Clinical features and practical diagnosis of bullous pemphigoid. Dermatol Clin 2011;29:427–38, viii-ix.
37. Fleming TE, Korman NJ. Cicatricial pemphigoid. J Am Acad Dermatol 2000;43: 571–91 [quiz: 91–4].

Erosive Lichen Planus

Melissa Mauskar, MD

KEYWORDS

- Erosive lichen planus • Vulva • Mucosal lichen planus • Scaring

KEY POINTS

- Erosive lichen planus is a painful, scaring condition of the vulva, oral mucosa, and rarely other mucous membranes.
- Untreated, lichen planus can lead to vaginal stenosis, vulvar agglutination, and rarely squamous cell carcinoma of non–hair-barring skin.
- Topical treatment helps most patients, but systemic therapy may be needed for severe disease.

INTRODUCTION

Lichen planus is a T-cell–mediated chronic inflammatory mucocutaneous condition with a myriad of clinical manifestations. Erosive lichen planus is an uncommon, painful condition of mucous membranes that leads to irreversible scaring when left untreated and can rarely progress to squamous cell carcinoma (SCC).[1] The oral mucosa is the most common site of involvement, and genital mucosa is the second most common area affected.[2] Taking a thorough past medical history and detailed physical examination is imperative; when any variant of lichen planus is suspected, a total body skin examination, including all mucosal areas, hair, and nails, should be performed. Aggressive early management with potent topical steroids often improves symptoms, but patients may require more than one treatment modality to prevent long-term sequelae. Patients with erosive lichen planus will require long-term management by a multidisciplinary team to optimize outcomes.

PATIENT HISTORY

The importance of taking a thorough history cannot be overemphasized. Although patients may present only for vulvar concerns, other mucosal sites are often involved; providers should ask for a complete review of symptoms.

Vulvar Disease

In one review, more than 92% of patients presented with burning or pain, whereas itch was found in 50%.[3] Both acute and chronic erosions of lichen planus can lead to

Department of Dermatology, UT Southwestern Medical Center at Dallas, 5323 Harry Hines Boulevard #MC-9190, Dallas, TX 75390-7208, USA
E-mail address: melissa.mauskar@utsouthwestern.edu

Obstet Gynecol Clin N Am 44 (2017) 407–420
http://dx.doi.org/10.1016/j.ogc.2017.04.004
0889-8545/17/© 2017 Elsevier Inc. All rights reserved.

dyspareunia, dysuria, or pain with defecation. Copious vaginal discharge, vulvar soreness, or difficulty urinating are other chief complaints. Unfortunately, these symptoms may be incorrectly attributed to candidiasis for years before a correct diagnosis is made.[4]

Patients may try various home remedies to alleviate their symptoms before seeking help from a provider; this may complicate the clinical picture, especially if patients use benzocaine or other numbing agents. These agents may lead to allergic contact dermatitis and even secondary ulcers or erosions. At the first visit patients should bring a list of everything they use in the vulvar area: topical medications, over-the-counter creams, soaps, douches, and lubricants.

Oral Disease

The oral cavity is the most common site of involvement of lichen planus.

Oral lesions precede genital lesions in one-third of patients; the conditions occur simultaneously in almost half of patients.[2] Patients may be asymptomatic or present with intractable burning or pain, inability to eat acidic foods, bleeding gums, swelling, or irritation. They may be diagnosed with oral lichen planus by their dentist but not associate this with current vulvar symptoms.

Other Mucosal Sites

The esophageal, ocular, and otic mucosa can rarely be involved and are likely under recognized. Therefore, all patients with documented erosive lichen planus should be screened for dysphagia, hearing loss, dry eye, or blurred vision. Like vulvar disease, if left untreated, these can lead to scarring and significant damage.

Psychosocial History

Patients with erosive lichen planus often exhibit signs of depression and poor quality of life and note impact on sexual functioning.[5,6] Providers should screen for these complications and consider referral to mental health experts when creating management strategies.

PHYSICAL EXAMINATION

It is not uncommon for patients to delay presentation for years because of anxiety and embarrassment. When this occurs, late-stage scaring and loss of normal architecture can obscure diagnosis (**Fig. 1**). When patients present with vulvar pain and burning, lichen planus should be on the differential diagnosis before entering the examination room. After a detailed vulvovaginal examination is done, and lichen planus is suspected, other commonly affected areas should also be examined.

Vulvovaginal Examination

Patients should be positioned in stirrups for a proper and thorough examination. There are 3 types of lichen planus that occur on the vulva: papulosquamous (**Fig. 2**), hypertrophic, and erosive. Erosive lichen planus is the most common subtype on the vulva.[6] Characteristic features of erosive lichen planus include well-demarcated pink-red erosions (**Fig. 3**), often with a white hyperkeratotic linear border or surrounding Wickham striae (**Fig. 4**). Erosions and inflammatory skin changes are most often seen at the introitus (90%), followed by vagina (20%–38%), vulva (37%), and perianal skin (8%).[7,8] These erosions may be difficult to appreciate for some providers. Careful examination of the vulva will reveal subtle changes in color or texture: take your time. Providers that are rushed during this step may miss an early clue to erosive lichen

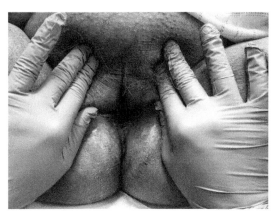

Fig. 1. Late-stage scaring and loss of normal architecture due to delayed presentation can obscure diagnosis.

planus that will save patients years of suffering. If needed, probing the vulvar skin with a Q-tip may help find the affected area.

Patients with late-stage disease can develop significant scarring, labia and clitoral hood resorption, complete burying of the clitoris, agglutination, strictures, synechiae, and in some cases complete fusion of the labia majora and stenosis of the vaginal introitus.[7–9]

After the vulva has been evaluated and no obvious adhesions or strictures are found, a vaginal examination should be done. The walls of the vaginal canal may have erythema, erosions, bleeding, or friable tissue. Late-stage disease may cause significant vaginal involvement prohibiting and even a small speculum to be advanced through the canal.[9] Wet mounts should always be done in patients suspected to have erosive lichen planus. Abundant parabasal cells and inflammation are clues to vaginal involvement and should not be overlooked.

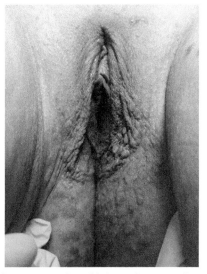

Fig. 2. Classic pruritic violaceous papules of lichen planus on the vulva.

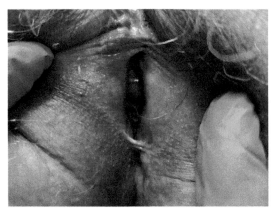

Fig. 3. Characteristic features of erosive lichen planus include well-demarcated pink-red erosions. Late stage agglutination is also seen.

Currently there is not a validated severity score of lichen planus. Providers should document the extent, location, and severity of lesions. Scaring should be quantified and described in a detailed manner. Photographs or drawings should be added to the medical record to help document the response to treatment.

Oral Examination

An oral examination should be performed on all patients who present with vulvar pain and burning, especially those suspected to have erosive lichen planus. Adequate lighting with abundant natural light (when available) in addition to focused overhead, flashlight, or gooseneck lamp will enable providers to detect subtle changes in color and texture. Gloved fingers and a tongue depressor should be used to visualize the cutaneous and mucosal lip, gingiva and gingival sulcus, tongue, hard and soft palate, and buccal mucosa. The most common site of involvement is the buccal mucosa, followed by the tongue, and gingiva. There are 3 major clinical forms: reticular, erythematous, and erosive.[2] Reticular pattern most often presents as asymptomatic white reticular lacy changes on the buccal mucosa. This finding should not be confused with morcicotio buccarum, a hyperkeratotic linear white plaque on buccal mucosa,

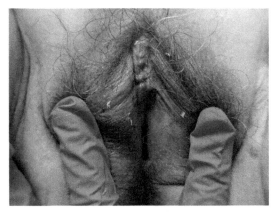

Fig. 4. Features of erosive lichen planus often include, agglutination of the labia minora and phymosis of the clitoral hood, violaceous patches with a white linear border.

a frequent finding in patients that grind their teeth at night or bite the inner cheeks. Gingival erosions, desquamative gingivitis, and violaceous plaques with overlying Wickham striae (**Fig. 5**) may also be found. Oral lichen planus is usually bilateral and symmetric; often more than one clinical subtype can be present at once.[2]

Other Common Locations

Common cutaneous sites of involvement, eyes, and ears should also be examined. Cutaneous lichen planus has a flexural predominance; the most frequent locations include wrists and forearms, neck, inguinal folds, and anterior legs. Seventeen percent to 22% of patients with erosive lichen planus may have concurrent cutaneous disease.[6] These lesions characteristically present as purple, polygonal, flat-toped papules that are pruritic and have overlying, fine white scales known as Wickham striae. Lichen planus is known to koebnerize or develop in areas of trauma.

Patients with ocular lichen planus will have injected sclera and conjunctival erosions and can process to blindness due to conjunctival scaring. Early referral to an experienced ophthalmologist is essential for these patients.[10] Although rare, otic involvement can lead to conductive hearing loss. Examination of the external ear canal may demonstrate erythema, induration, and stenosis.[11]

Patients with erosive lichen planus will often need a multidisciplinary team of clinicians; referrals to specialists should not be delayed.

Additional Testing: Biopsy

Patients may present at different stages of erosive disease, including early, when there is only a hint of color change signifying a new erosion; established lesions, well demarcated with a white treadlike border; or late, when severe scaring is well underway.

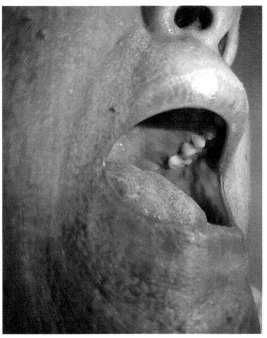

Fig. 5. Features of oral lichen planus include violaceous plaques with overlying Wickham striae at gingival margins.

Late-stage erosive lichen planus may be impossible to distinguish from lichen sclerosis or mucous membrane pemphigoid; therefore, a biopsy is required for proper diagnosis.

Where should you biopsy? Location is vital to a proper diagnosis. White reticular boarders are often the best places to biopsy. If ulcerations are present, biopsy should include half of the erosion and half normal skin. If a biopsy is done in the center of the erosion, the pathologist may not be able to distinguish erosive lichen planus from other scaring conditions of the vulva. A shave biopsy is usually adequate for tissue collection.

When filling out the pathology form, it is important to give as much clinical history as possible. Providing detailed information, such as *45-year-old woman with vulvar pain and superficial erosions*, will generate a better clinicopathologic correlation than writing, *vulvar lesion*.

Histopathology

The hallmark of lichen planus is a lichenoid interface dermatitis and dense bandlike lymphocytic infiltrate often extending from the dermal-epidermal junction to the upper reticular dermis; this infiltrate may obliterate the basal layer of the epidermis. Other features include irregular acanthosis of the epidermis, liquefactive degeneration of the basal cell layer, and sawtooth pattern of the rete ridges.[2,12] Erosive lichen planus may lack characteristic findings seen in cutaneous lichen planus and may be nonspecific. It is important to have a dermatopathologist review biopsies for the best clinicopathologic correlation, as noted earlier.

Diagnostic Criteria

Recently, diagnostic criteria for erosive lichen planus affecting the vulva were reached through an electronic-Delphi consensus pooling members of the International Society for the Study of Vulvovaginal Disease.[13] Nine diagnostic criteria were viewed as essential for the diagnosis of erosive lichen planus (**Box 1**). Three of out of the 9 criteria are required for the diagnosis of erosive lichen planus of the vulva.

Box 1
Diagnostic criteria for erosive lichen planus affecting the vulva

Presence of well-demarcated erosions or glazed erythema at the vaginal introitus

Presence of a hyperkeratotic white border to erythematous areas/erosions ± Wickham striae in surrounding skin

Symptoms of pain/burning

Scarring/loss of normal architecture

Presence of vaginal inflammation

Involvement of other mucosal sites

Presence of a well-defined inflammatory band in the superficial connective tissue that involves the dermoepidermal junction

Presence of an inflammatory band that consists predominantly of lymphocytes

Signs of basal cell layer degeneration, for example, Civatte bodies, abnormal keratinocytes, or basal apoptosis

From Simpson RC, Thomas KS, Leighton P, et al. Diagnostic criteria for erosive lichen planus affecting the vulva: an international electronic-Delphi consensus exercise. Br J Dermatol 2013;169(2):342; with permission.

PHARMACOLOGIC TREATMENT OPTIONS

The treatment and management of patients with erosive lichen planus are challenging. Goals of care are aimed at improving symptoms and halting disease progression. Experts agree that topical steroids should be used as the first-line treatment; however, 25% to 40% of patients respond poorly to topical treatment and will require systemic therapy.[8,13,14] Large prospective randomized controlled trials on vulvar erosive lichen planus are lacking, as evidenced by a recent Cochrane review on mucosal lichen planus excluding studies of genital disease.[15,16]

Local Treatment

Topical corticosteroids

Ultrapotent, class I topical steroids like clobetasol 0.05% ointment and augmented betamethasone dipropionate 0.05% are first-line treatments for erosive lichen planus. In the only prospective study of 114 patients with erosive vulvar lichen planus, 94% reported symptomatic improvement and 71% were symptom free after twice-daily application of clobetasol for 3 months.[14]

A second study noted 55% of patients responded to topical steroids alone for induction therapy and symptomatic improvement of disease.[7] Ointments are always the preferred vehicles over creams for vulvar skin; creams contain alcohol and preservatives that will burn when applied to open erosions.

Patients should use ultrapotent steroids once to twice a day for 1 month and then return to the office for evaluation. At that time, many patients will note improvement in symptoms. Daily application may need to be continued for up to 3 months; but once symptoms improve, therapy should be tapered slowly, either by lowering the strength or by decreasing application as possible.

At the initial visit, patients should be educated about how much and where to apply their topical medication. This instruction can be done in the office with patients holding a hand mirror and petroleum jelly (Vaseline) as a test vehicle. Topical steroids should only be used on affected areas of non–hair-bearing skin. Patients should apply a small pea-sized amount and should not feel greasy or sticky after applying the medication. At the conclusion of the visit, patients should receive a diagram, photograph, or detailed instructions on where to apply their medication to limit side effects. Emollients like Vaseline or Aquaphor should not be underestimated; these can be used between topical steroid application to protect against urine and other agents that may exacerbate symptoms. Secondary infections, such as candidiasis or herpes simplex, can occur; thus, patients should be seen in the clinic if they report worsening of disease.

Intralesional triamcinolone acetonide (Kenalog) injections are quite helpful for stubborn lesions. Concentrations of 5 to 10 mg/mL should be used in the affected area. An injection of 0.1 mL of Kenalog will diffuse approximately 1 cm^2 in the tissue, allowing clinicians to estimate the amount needed to treat a particular area.[17] Injections should be given every 3 to 4 weeks based on the response to treatment and may provide significant benefit. Patients should be warned of the side effects of this treatment, such as mucosal atrophy, scaring, hypopigmentation, or infection. Should lesions not resolve, institution of systemic agents should not be delayed.

Topical calcineurin inhibitors

There are several reports demonstrating tacrolimus 0.1% ointment twice daily to be an effective topical treatment of both oral and genital erosive lichen planus.[7,9,18–20] This agent is a steroid-sparing agent that is approved by the Food and Drug Administration (FDA) for atopic dermatitis in adults and children greater than 2 years of age. Application to friable and eroded tissue can cause irritation in some patients; thus, it may prove a better agent for maintenance therapy. Additionally, topical tacrolimus does not have the side effects (atrophy, erythema, telangiectasias) of topical steroids.

Systemic treatments

There are a variety of oral therapies used for erosive lichen planus (**Table 1**). Currently, there are no randomized control trials comparing systemic therapy for erosive genital lichen planus. The 4 most common agents used include prednisone, methotrexate, mycophenolate mofetil, and hydroxychloroquine.[8] Other anecdotal agents include rituximab,[21] cyclosporine,[22] tacrolimus,[23] minocycline, and niacinamide[8] and were found to be helpful in some cases. Each agent will require laboratory monitoring and close follow-up for their respective side effects.

There is a randomized control trial on the horizon. Rosalind and colleagues[24] published a protocol for the hELP trial, whereby they plan to analyze the 4 most common agents used: prednisone, methotrexate, mycophenolate mofetil, and hydroxychloroquine.

Corticosteroids

Prednisone is the agent of choice for many providers when patients have disease flares or are not responding appropriately to topical therapy. Daily morning doses ranging from 40 to 60 mg for 2 to 4 weeks notably improves erosive lichen planus.[9] Prednisone provides significant relief for patients but should almost never be considered a maintenance therapy because of the significant long-term side effects.

Methotrexate

Methotrexate has been reported to be a relatively safe and effective long-term systemic agent for erosive lichen planus. Baseline complete blood cell count, liver function tests, urinalysis, hepatitis panel, and creatine should be ordered before treatment commences. Patients with high alcohol intake or propensity for fatty liver disease should be screened before starting this treatment, as long-term use can accelerate cirrhosis of the liver. A test dose of 5 mg is often prescribed and slowly titrated according to the response to a maximum of 25 mg/wk. Patients should take daily folic acid supplementation to reduce side effects. The most severe side effect of methotrexate is pancytopenia, often from patients incorrectly taking tablets daily instead of doses weekly.

Mycophenolate mofetil

Mycophenolate mofetil (MMF) is started at 500 mg once daily and slowly titrated up to a maximum dosage of 1.5 g twice daily. This medication can cause significant gastrointestinal distress, and patients should take this medication with meals if possible. Although there are several reports of oral erosive lichen planus improving with MMF, large studies of genital disease are lacking. One case report of MMF in a 66-year-old patient noted significant improvement after 4 months of treatment of 500 mg in the morning and 1 g at night. MMF has a relatively low side effect profile compared with other steroid-sparing agents and is frequently used as a maintenance therapy in other autoimmune and inflammatory disorders in dermatology.[25]

Hydroxychloroquine

Hydroxychloroquine has been noted to be beneficial for treatment of oral lichen planus. Typically, treatment is started at 200 mg twice daily; but effects may be delayed for 2 to 3 months of therapy.[9] Several experts note that this therapy is not as effective for genital disease; however, large studies are lacking.[7]

Table 1
Systemic treatment of erosive lichen planus

Drug	Dose	Laboratory Tests to Follow	Mechanism	Side Effects	Interactions
Prednisone (1, 2, 5, 10, 20, 50 mg)	40–60 mg	If long-term therapy (>3 mo of >20 mg/d); BP, PPD, DEXA; Ca++ supplement (1000 mg/vitD 800 IU) and bisphosphonate	Decreases AP-1, cyclooxygenase, NF-KB; decreases proinflammatory cytokines (especially IL-2)	Hyperglycemia, insomnia, HTN, infection, osteoporosis, avascular necrosis, cataracts, adrenal insufficiency, peptic ulcer, poor wound healing	metabolized by CYP3A4
Methotrexate 2.5 mg	Begin at 5 mg–25 mg qwk **w/folate 1 mg qd	Baseline CBC, CMP, hepatitis panel F/U: CBC/LFTs qwk ×4 then q3mo	Inhibits dihydrofolate reductase; cell-cycle specific (S phase)	Hepatotoxic, cancer, bone marrow depression, pulmonary fibrosis/ pneumonitis, alopecia, UV recall	EtOH, NSAIDs, TCNs, retinoids, TMP/SMX, dapsone
Mycophenolate mofetil (CellCept 500 mg)	0.5–1.5 g bid	Baseline: CBC, LFTs F/U: CBC qwk ×4 then qmo + LFTs qmo	Inhibits inosine monophosphate dehydrogenase → de novo purine biosynthesis	GI symptoms (Myfortic = enteric coated, less GI effects), BM depression, hepatotoxicity	Cholestyramine, iron, mag/al, acyclovir
Cyclosporine 25/100 mg	Start at 2.5 mg/kg/d max 5 mg 1 y max	Baseline, q2wk (then qmo): CBC, BMP, LFTs, FLP, Mg, Uric acid, BP	Binds cyclophilin → inhibits calcineurin activation of NF-AT; inhibits IL-2, IFN gamma	*Nephrotoxic, HTN* (use CCB, no ACE/diuretic), low magnesium, high potassium, hyperlipidemia, cancer, ha, acne, uricemia	Metabolized by CYP34a, grapefruit juice, methotrexate, SSRI
Hydroxychloroquine (Plaquenil) 200 mg	200 mg twice daily	Baseline: eye examination, CBC	All antimalarials: intercalate into DNA preventing transcription, inhibit IL-2	Blue pigment, GI upset, retinopathy (peripheral fields), psoriasis	Cimetidine, digoxin, kaolin, mg
Rituximab (Rituxan)	RA: 1 g on day 1, then day 15; repeat at 6 mo if relapse	Baseline: CBC, hepatitis panel, HIV, q6–12mo	Anti-CD20 monoclonal antibody	Infusion rxn, JC virus infx, severe mucocutaneous reactions	None

Abbreviations: ACE, angiotensin-converting enzyme; BP, blood pressure; CBC, complete blood cell count; F/U, follow-up; GI, gastrointestinal; HIV, human immunodeficiency virus; HTN, hypertension; IFN, interferon; IL, interleukin; LFTs, liver function tests; max, maximum; NSAIDs, nonsteroidal antiinflammatory drugs; SSRI, selective serotonin reuptake inhibitor; vitD, vitamin D.

Naturopathic therapies Some patients may want to avoid prescription medications in favor of a more holistic approach. Two recent studies show promising results for oral lichen planus and may prove useful for genital disease as well.

Oral curcuminoids Turmeric is a natural spice used for thousands of years in both the culinary industry and Ayurvedic medicine; it is thought to be a potent antiinflammatory agent. A recent study lends strong support for use of the active ingredient of turmeric, oral curcuminoids, for treating oral lichen planus.[26] High-dose curcuminoids at a dosage of 6000 mg/d in 3 divided doses were used in this study of 20 patients. Compared with controls, patients on the oral curcuminoids had a statistically significant decrease in erythema and ulceration. Although this is a small sample size, it may warrant a treatment trial as there are little to no side effects noted to date; anecdotally, many patients have improved on this therapy along with topical antiinflammatories.

Zinc

A recent study reviewed the systemic zinc levels in patients with oral erosive lichen planus, nonerosive lichen planus, and controls. Patients with oral erosive lichen planus were noted to have statistically lower zinc levels than the other two groups, postulating that zinc supplementation may improve wound healing and increase reepithelization.[27] Zinc deficiency is noted to cause acquired acrodermatitis enteropathica, a nutritional deficiency with significant erosions in the oral, perianal, and genital skin.

NONPHARMACOLOGIC TREATMENT OPTIONS

There are increasing reports in the literature evaluating novel treatment options for lichen planus.

Photodynamic Therapy

Photodynamic therapy (PDT) is an FDA-approved treatment of precancerous lesions and some types of basal cell carcinoma. A light-sensitizing agent, such as aminolevulinic acid (ALA), methyl 5-aminolevulinate, or hexyl 5-aminolevulinate hydrochloride (HAL), is applied to the lesion and allowed to incubate. Next, patients are exposed to a red or blue light to activate the treatment. Several studies, most done in Europe, have investigated HAL-PDT for vulvar erosive lichen planus.[28,29] Helgesen and colleagues[29] developed a randomized control trial comparing HAL-PDT with topical corticosteroids over a 48-week period. The mean reduction of itch and pain was similar in the PDT group compared with the corticosteroid group. At 6 weeks' follow-up, there were no significant differences between treatment groups; however, patients in the PDT group reported using less topical steroids from week 7 to 24. Limitations to this study include low sample size (20 patients in each group) and the treatment group requiring general anesthesia during treatment secondary to pain.[28] There are additional reports of ALA-PDT used for papulosquamous genital lichen planus lesions with a good response rate.[30]

LASER THERAPY

One study of carbon dioxide (CO_2) laser treatment of clitoral phimosis due to lichen sclerosus or lichen planus has been reported to date. Twenty patients with lichen sclerosis and 3 with lichen planus were treated; however, 2 of the patients with lichen planus required reoperation after treatment.[31] There are several reports of refractory oral erosive lichen planus lesions successfully treated with CO_2 laser.[32]

COMBINATION THERAPIES

Many patients will require a combination of topical and oral treatment, with topical steroids and prednisone/methotrexate sited as the most effective treatment regimens for genital disease.

One retrospective study of 131 patients with erosive lichen planus showed promising results with a combination therapy of ultrapotent topical steroids and methotrexate or low-dose prednisolone.[7] Initial disease control was obtained with either oral or topical corticosteroids. After symptomatic control and resolution of inflammatory changes and erosions was achieved, patients were switched to topical tacrolimus, if tolerated. Patients who developed flares when oral prednisolone was tapered were started on methotrexate weekly plus daily folic acid 5 mg. All compliant patients achieved objective and symptomatic disease control in a mean of 7.5 weeks. A large proportion, 48 of 131 of those patients (37%), required multimodal therapy to maintain their initial improvement.[7]

TREATMENT RESISTANCE AND COMPLICATIONS

Unfortunately, treatment resistance is not uncommon. Prolonged topical steroid use may predispose patients to side effects, such as erythema, striae, and secondary infections. Proper application should be reviewed frequently to avoid these unwanted side effects.

Although symptoms may improve, vaginal disease can progress leading to vaginal wall adhesion, scaring, and strictures. In fact, in 114 patients only 50% reported improvement in vulvar erosions after topical steroid application and only 9% had complete clinical remission of clinical signs.[14] Late-stage disease can prohibit penetrative intercourse and cause difficulty urinating. When this occurs, surgical adhesion of strictures and synechiae may be the only option to restore these functions.

SURGICAL TREATMENT OPTIONS

Once adhesions or syncytia develop, surgical separation by a gynecologist experienced in treatment of vulvar and vaginal lichen planus is necessary. This procedure often occurs in an operating room while patients are anesthetized. One technique by Fairchild and Haefner[33] has good results, with 95% of patients feeling satisfied with their procedure. To summarize this technique, superficial adhesions are separated mechanically with betadine-soaked sponge sticks, while both sharp and blunt dissection are required for late-stage stenosis. Once the desired length and width of the vagina is achieved, a foam dilator covered with sterile condoms is placed in the vagina for 48 hours. The dilator is removed in follow-up, and patients are placed on high-dose intravaginal steroids. Patients should be counseled that there will be significant postoperative clinic follow-up, along with lifelong home dilator use and intravaginal steroids to maintain patency of the vagina.

EVALUATION OF OUTCOME AND LONG-TERM RECOMMENDATIONS

Both disease activity and symptoms must be targeted and controlled. Unfortunately, erosive lichen planus is a chronic condition that can be very difficult to manage. Goals of treatment and expectations should be established early in the physician-patient relationship. As evidenced earlier, many different treatment options and modalities may be used before an effective regimen is established.

Individualization of treatment regimens remains a mainstay of treatment. In one study of 131 patients, 48 (37%) required multiple agents to control both symptoms and disease progression.[7] At long-term follow-up, 88 (77%) patients reported symptom control and no progressive tissue destruction, whereas 27 (23%) patients had unstable symptom control and progressive tissue destruction.[7]

DEVELOPMENT OF SQUAMOUS CELL CARCINOMA

Risk of SCC in lichen planus depends on the location of involvement. Lichen planus on extragenital skin has no cancer risk, but oral and esophageal involvement has been reported as 5%.[1] In a recent article analyzing the development of SCC in patients with vulvar lichen planus, one-third arose in erosive disease, with the other two-thirds developing papules and plaques. All lesions were located on non–hair-bearing vulvar mucosa.[1]

The malignant transformation rate of erosive lichen planus is reported to be 2.3% in one study; however, large-scale prospective studies are lacking.[8] Lichen planus–associated SCCs are aggressive malignancies; at presentation, there is a high rate of regional lymph node metastases. More than 30% of disease-related deaths are reported within the first 1 to 3 years after diagnosis. Within the first 12 months of diagnosis of SCC, almost 40% of patients had recurrent cancer in residual lichen planus lesions.[1] Regular follow-up is imperative to long-term successful outcomes.

Monitoring Guidelines

Patients with erosive lichen planus should be followed regularly every 6 months to prevent and monitor for development of SCC. The vulva, mons pubis, and introitus should be evaluated for development of hyperkeratotic plaque, ulcerated papules, glistening red thickened plaques, or tumors obliterating existing architecture. When SCC is suspected, patients should be examined for palpable inguinal lymphadenopathy. Punch biopsies should be taken for suspicious lesions to ensure depth is adequately sampled.

Impact on Quality of Life

Erosive lichen planus is a chronic and painful condition that women often suffer with for months (even years) before presenting to a physician for evaluation. In one study, 69% of women with erosive lichen planus of the vulva reported sexual distress. Women with erosive lichen planus have a worse reported quality of life than those with lichen sclerosus.[5,8] Providers should take this into consideration when treating and managing patients with erosive lichen planus; patients may need referral to sexual counselors, psychologists, or psychiatrists for holistic treatment.

Vulvodynia

Once initial symptoms have improved and disease progression has abated with treatment, some patients may note increased pain; it is not uncommon for patients with prior vulvar disease, especially erosive lichen planus, to develop vulvodynia. Both conditions should be addressed and treated, and patients should be counseled on topical and oral neuromodulating treatments to help with their vulvar pain.

SUMMARY

Erosive lichen planus is a chronic, painful, scaring, and emotionally disabling condition. Symptoms are greatly improved with topical steroids, but multimodal treatment may be required to prevent progressive architectural changes. Patients must be monitored regularly to assess for treatment modifications and progression of disease. Creation of a clinical severity score for erosive lichen planus in conjunction with large-scale randomized control studies are needed to determine optimal treatment algorithms and assess clinical outcome measures.

REFERENCES

1. Regauer S, Reich O, Eberz B. Vulvar cancers in women with vulvar lichen planus: a clinicopathological study. J Am Acad Dermatol 2014;71(4):698–707.
2. Olson MA, Rodgers RA, Bruse AJ. Oral lichen planus. Clin Dermatol 2016;34(4): 495–504.
3. Cheng H, Oakley A, Rowan D, et al. Diagnostic criteria in 72 women with erosive vulvovaginal lichen planus. Australas J Dermatol 2016;57(4):284–7.
4. Machin SE, McConnell DT, Adams JD. Vaginal lichen planus: preservation of sexual function in severe disease. BMJ Case Rep 2010;2010 [pii:bcr08.2009.2208].
5. Cheng H, Oakley A, Conaglen J, et al. Quality of life and sexual distress in women with erosive vulvovaginal lichen planus. J Low Genit Tract Dis 2016;21(2):145–9.
6. Gorouhi F, Davari P, Fazel N. Cutaneous and mucosal lichen planus: a comprehensive review of clinical subtypes, risk factors, diagnosis, and prognosis. ScientificWorldJournal 2014;2014:742826.
7. Bradford J, Fischer G. Management of vulvovaginal lichen planus: a new approach. J Low Genit Tract Dis 2013;17(1):28–32.
8. Simpson RC, Littlewood SM, Cooper SM, et al. Real-life experience of managing vulval erosive lichen planus: a case-based review and U.K. multicenter case note audit. Br J Dermatol 2012;167(1):85–91.
9. Moyal-Barracco M, Edwards L. Diagnosis and therapy of anogenital lichen planus. Dermatol Ther 2004;17:38–46.
10. Pakravan M, Klesert TR, Akpek EK. Isolated lichen planus of the conjunctiva. Br J Ophthalmol 2006;90(10):1325–6.
11. Sartori-Valinotti JC, Bruce AJ, Khan YK, et al. A 10-year review of otic lichen planus the Mayo Clinic experience. JAMA Dermatol 2013;149(9):1082–6.
12. Shiohara T, Kano Y. Lichen planus and lichenoid dermatoses. In: Bolognia JL, Jorizzo JL, Schaffer JV, editors. Dermatology. 3rd edition. China: Elsevier Saunders; 2009. p. 183–202.
13. Simpson RC, Thomas KS, Leighton P, et al. Diagnostic criteria for erosive lichen planus affecting the vulva: an international electronic-Delphi consensus exercise. Br J Dermatol 2013;169(2):337–43.
14. Cooper SM, Wojnarowska S. Influence of treatment of erosive lichen planus of the vulva on its prognosis. Arch Dermatol 2006;142:289–94.
15. Lewis FM, Bogliatto F. Erosive vulval lichen planus—a diagnosis not to be missed: a clinical review. Eur J Obstet Gynecol Reprod Biol 2013;171:214–9.
16. Cheng S, Kirtschig G, Cooper S, et al. Interventions for erosive lichen planus affecting mucosal sites. Cochrane Database Syst Rev 2012;(2):CD008092.
17. Edwards L, Lynch P. Genital dermatology. Philadelphia: Lippincott Williams and Williams; 2011.
18. Byrd JA, Davis MD, Rogers RS. Recalcitrant symptomatic vulvar lichen planus: response to topical tacrolimus. Arch Dermatol 2004;140(6):715–20.
19. Jensen JT, Bird M, Leclair CM. Patient satisfaction after the treatment of vulvovaginal erosive lichen planus with topical clobetasol and tacrolimus: a survey study. Am J Obstet Gynecol 2004;190(6):1759–63 [discussion: 1763–5].

20. Goldstein AT, Thaçi D, Luger T. Topical calcineurin inhibitors for the treatment of vulvar dermatoses. Eur J Obstet Gynecol Reprod Biol 2009;146(1):22–9.
21. Heelan K, McAleer MA, Roche L, et al. Intractable erosive lichen planus treated successfully with rituximab. Br J Dermatol 2015;172(2):538–40.
22. Ho VC, Gupta AK, Ellis CN, et al. Treatment of severe lichen planus with cyclosporine. J Am Acad Dermatol 1990;22:64Y8.
23. Yeo L, Ormerod AD. Oral tacrolimus: a treatment option for recalcitrant erosive lichen planus. Clin Exp Dermatol 2016;41:680–91.
24. Rosalind C, Simpson RC, Murphy R, et al. Systemic therapy for vulval erosive lichen planus (the 'hELP' trial): study protocol for a randomised controlled trial. Trials 2016;17:2.
25. Deen K, Mcmeniman E. Mycophenolate mofetil in erosive genital lichen planus: a case and review of the literature. J Dermatol 2015;42:311–4.
26. Chainani-Wu N, Madden E, Lozada-Nur F, et al. High-dose curcuminoids are efficacious in the reduction in symptoms and signs of oral lichen planus. J Am Acad Dermatol 2012;66(5):752–60.
27. Gholizadeh NA, Mehdipour MB, Najafi SA, et al. Evaluation of the serum zinc level in erosive and non-erosive oral lichen planus. J Dent (Shiraz) 2014;15(2):52–6.
28. Wennberg AM. Vulvovaginal photodynamic therapy for genital erosive lichen planus. Br J Dermatol 2015;173(5):1119–20.
29. Helgesen AL, Warloe T, Pripp AH, et al. Vulvovaginal photodynamic therapy vs. topical corticosteroids in genital erosive lichen planus: a randomized controlled trial. Br J Dermatol 2015;173(5):1156–62.
30. Fan Z, Zhang L, Wang H, et al. Treatment of cutaneous lichen planus with ALA-mediated topical photodynamic therapy. J Innovative Opt Health Sci 2015;8(1):1–7.
31. Kroft J, Shier M. A novel approach to the surgical management of clitoral phimosis. J Obstet Gynaecol Can 2012;34(5):465–71.
32. Mahdavi O, Boostani N, Jajarm HH, et al. Use of low level laser therapy for oral lichen planus: report of two cases. J Dent (Shiraz) 2013;14(4):201–4.
33. Fairchild PS, Haefner HK. Surgical management of vulvovaginal agglutination due to lichen planus. Am J Obstet Gynecol 2016;214(2):289.e1-2.

Fissures, Herpes Simplex Virus, and Drug Reactions
Important Erosive Vulvar Disorders

Tanja G. Bohl, MBBS, FACD*

KEYWORDS

- Vulva • Erosions • Herpes simplex • Drug reactions • Immunocompetence

KEY POINTS

- Vulvar fissures, erosions, excoriations, and erosions are common problems resulting from a variety of etiologies, many involving other mucosal and cutaneous sites.
- We present historical and examination features and useful investigations that can help establish a diagnosis so that definitive therapy can be instituted.
- Vulvar involvement also can be part of life-threatening conditions that require hospital admission and a multidisciplinary approach for optimal patient care.
- The clinical morphology of these examination findings and response to therapy can be modified by various host factors, particularly immune status, and atypical presentations and responses to therapy should always prompt patient reevaluation.

GENERAL CONSIDERATIONS

Vulvar erosions and fissures (**Table 1**) are a common problem. This reflects their diverse range of etiologies, which include common activities exposing women to physical and chemical irritation as well as common dermatoses that may affect the vulva. Any cause of vulvar pruritus increases the likelihood of erosions and fissures as women scratch, rub, and apply various compounds and medicaments to reduce this symptom. These actions can increase the risk of infection and further damage the vulvar tissue. Differential diagnoses in any individual patient will depend on age, history, and presenting features. Differential diagnoses are arranged in **Box 1** in a manner to indicate the most common and important but more rare conditions.

Erosions are superficial lesions with partial loss of the epidermis that can be due to a variety of causes. These are usually painful, often multiple, and may coalesce resulting in large denuded areas with serous fluid exudate and crusting occurring to varying degrees. They may be the only type of lesion present or, depending on their etiology, may be present along with ulcers (complete loss of epidermis), flaccid bullae (uncommonly

Vulva Clinic, Jean Hailes Medical Centre, 173 Carinish Road, Clayton, Victoria 3168, Australia
* Clinic 41, 41 Monash Road, Newborough, Victoria 3825, Australia.
E-mail address: tanjabohl@bigpond.com

Obstet Gynecol Clin N Am 44 (2017) 421–443
http://dx.doi.org/10.1016/j.ogc.2017.05.005
0889-8545/17/© 2017 Published by Elsevier Inc.

obgyn.theclinics.com

Table 1
Vulvar lesion definitions

Lesion	Definition	Appearance
Erosion	Partial-thickness loss of epithelium, superficial	
Fissure	Linear loss of epidermis that is usually superficial but can be deep, in which case it becomes a linear ulcer	
Crust	Dried secretions from broken epithelium, including serous fluid, pus, blood, bacteria	
Excoriation	Break in the epithelium due to scratching or hard rubbing, usually partial thickness	
Ulcer	Full-thickness loss of epithelium, depth varies and can extend through full thickness of dermis	

Box 1
Causes of vulvar erosions and fissures

Infections
- Herpes Simplex 1 and 2
- Candidiasis
- Varicella zoster
- Human immunodeficiency virus
- Streptococcus (pediatric cases) (bullous impetigo)

Mechanical/Localized Tissue Damage
- Excoriations
- Tight clothing
- Sexual activity
- Bicycle riding/horse riding
- Intertrigo: obesity
- Undercleansing: urine, feces
- Overcleaning: rubbing, irritating chemicals

Dermatoses

Inflammatory
- Eczema; atopic, irritant, or contact dermatitis
- Psoriasis
- Seborrheic dermatitis
- Zinc deficiency (acquired): elderly, poorly nourished, post bariatric surgery
- Erythema multiforme majus
- Stevens-Johnson syndrome/toxic epidermal necrolysis
- Fixed drug eruption
- Graft-versus-host disease
- Lichen planus
- Lichen sclerosus

Autoimmune Vesiculobullous, Intraepidermal/Intraepithelial
- Pemphigus vulgaris
- Pemphigus vegetans
- Paraneoplastic pemphigus

Autoimmune Vesiculobullous, Subepidermal/Epithelial
- Bullous pemphigoid
- Mucous membrane pemphigoid
- Systemic lupus erythematosus
- Linear immunoglobulin A disease

Inherited
- Benign familial pemphigus/Hailey-Hailey
- Darier disease
- Zinc deficiency: acrodermatitis enteropathica

---

seen even in bullous diseases of the vulva due to their superficial nature), pustules, vesicles, or other morphologies. Rupture of these lesions may cause erosions and, depending on when a patient presents for consultation, the primary and more diagnostic clinical features, such as vesicles or intraepidermal bullae, may be lost. The occurrence of infection of erosive lesions can result in further tissue loss causing ulcers. Ulcers involve full-thickness loss of the epidermis. Fissures are linear lesions and may be superficial (erosions) or deep (ulcers). Superficial fissures can be difficult to see on clinical examination, either because they are small and narrow or because they may be intermittent in nature and thus not present on physical examination at the time of clinical evaluation, and the severity of fissures also may be more substantial than appreciated on a casual glance without careful examination and palpation of the tissue.

A careful and structured history that includes details of the lesions, the general skin and mucous membranes, medications taken for any reason not just to treat or alleviate their vulvar conditions, gynecologic, reproductive, contraceptive, the general health of the patient and a familial history are an important foundation to establishing a diagnosis (**Box 2**).

The age of the patient and hormonal status of the patient also will influence what diagnoses are more likely. Irritant contact dermatitis due to urinary incontinence is more likely in a postmenopausal woman, herpes simplex infections are more likely to be in the reproductive years, and most heritable disorders will present within the first or second decade.

Box 2
Key questions

Primary symptom/presenting problem?
- Initial symptom(s) and if this has changed since onset
- Time between onset of symptoms and examination

Any associated changes?
- Genital; vaginal discharge, dyspareunia/apareunia
- Extragenital; constitution prodrome of fever, malaise, headache; other mucosal involvement: oral, ocular

Is this the first time this has occurred?

What has been done to improve the situation; self or medically instigated?
- Note any oral or topical agents or activities (additional cleansing)

Details of vulvar care and if this has altered
- Cleansing technique; cleansers, wipes, panty liners or other sanitary products

Medication history
- Generally used
- Specific to the presenting problem; topical and oral

General medical history
- Diabetes
- Autoimmune disorders
- Immune status
- Nutritional history; "natural" supplements may not be considered "medication," but can cause drug eruptions

Dermatologic history
- Genital and extragenital dermatoses

Sexual history
- History of sexually transmitted diseases
- New partner(s)
- Contraceptive use; condoms

Gynecologic history
- Hormonal status
- Continence
- Cervical cytology history
- Parity
- Past procedures
- Past illnesses

Familial history
- Any similar conditions
- Autoimmune diseases

The clinician's eyes, appreciation of normal anatomy, and how this may vary with age and a careful history are the most essential tools to establishing a preliminary diagnosis and arranging additional investigations, as in **Box 3**, to help finalize a diagnosis.

Box 3
Diagnostic tools to establish and finalize diagnosis

Examination tools

- Good source of lighting
- General examination couch or gynecologic couch
- Speculae (vaginal examination may not be possible in erosive disorders because of pain)
- Equipment for taking microbiologic specimens
  - General microbiologic cultures
  - Polymerase chain reaction swabs for viral DNA testing
  - Sabouraud media for direct plating for fungal culture (the appropriateness of testing for sexually transmissible diseases should be considered on an individual basis)
  - Glass slides and coverslips; unfixed slide of swab material for microscopy offsite (when wet mount not done)
- Wet mount; loop for collecting discharge, glass slide and coverslips and microscope
- Saline to cleanse discharge and enable visualization of structures

Biopsy

- Topical and injectable local anesthetic
- Punch biopsy in 3-mm, 4-mm, 5-mm, and 6-mm sizes, according to condition
- Monsel paste for hemostasis or dissolvable suture for wound closure
- Aftercare patient information sheet
- Specimen jars with 40% formalin for histopathology and transport media for direct immunofluorescence

Colposcopy

- "Vulvoscopy" is not essential, although the colposcope does provide a source of lighting and magnification

Blood Investigations

- Full blood examination and differential examination (possible blood dyscrasias, eosinophilia)
- Liver function tests
- Renal function tests
- Indirect immunofluorescence
- Antinuclear factor and extractable nuclear antigen
- Serology for sexually transmitted disease including human immunodeficiency virus
- Serum zinc
- HLA studies (possibly in future)/currently available in some institutions

Other Investigations

- Patch testing
- Prick testing

A requested consultation in the emergency department or inpatient setting will require a different approach to one referred to an outpatient clinic with a more chronic or recurrent problem. Questionnaires are becoming an increasingly popular way in which to ensure a thorough history. This approach is more suited to the latter. Readers are advised to have in mind all the areas to consider but ask a presentation-oriented series of questions modified to the patient in front of them.

The clinical examination should be thorough and include other body sites that may provide additional diagnostic information, such as other mucosal sites. In particular, the entire ano-genital area should be examined, including the inguinal creases and natal cleft. A vaginal examination may be required, but the general comfort of the patient and sexual maturity should be considered before proceeding. Analgesia may be required to enable an examination to be conducted. Application of acetic acid should not be done if there are erosions or fissures present because this is very painful.

Refer to colleagues if other mucosal sites are involved or if there is generalized involvement or suspicion of a drug reaction whereby alternative medication will be required, such as antiepileptic therapy.

A biopsy is not always required to finalize a diagnosis; however, if performed, it should be taken from the edge of an erosion or adjacent tissue or both. Specimens should be sent for general histologic examination and direct immunofluorescence. The biopsy site should be taken from the area most likely to give the greatest amount of information.

Blood tests again will be of value in certain suspected diagnoses and their use considered on an individual-patient basis. Serology for herpes simplex virus is not currently indicated for patient assessment[1], similarly the role of HLA testing is improving our understanding of the pathophysiology of drug eruptions but is not part of the assessment of patients with drug eruptions.

FISSURES

Vulvar fissures are linear erosions that generally can be classified into 2 main clinical groups:

- Splitting at the posterior fourchette "the 6 o'clock split" (**Fig. 1**)
- Splits/fissures within interlabial sulci and other skin folds

Splitting at the Posterior Fourchette

The mechanism of fissures at the posterior fourchette is often unknown. The usual history is one of splitting at the "6 o'clock" position during intercourse with pain on contact with seminal fluid, urine, or toilet tissue being the most common symptom. The clinical examination may reproduce the splitting on "tenting" of the posterior fourchette.

The term "membranous hypertrophy of the posterior fourchette" has been coined to describe this observation and it is considered a normal variant.[2]

If relief cannot be achieved with increased lubrication during intercourse and possibly modified sexual positions, surgery to enlarge the introitus (perineoplasty) has been successful in some cases. Medical therapy should be maximized first and demonstrate failure before surgical treatment is considered.

Topical estrogen or corticosteroid preparations have not been consistently shown to be beneficial unless a nonmechanical cause is contributing to fissure development; for example, estrogen deficiency, atopic dermatitis, or lichen sclerosus.

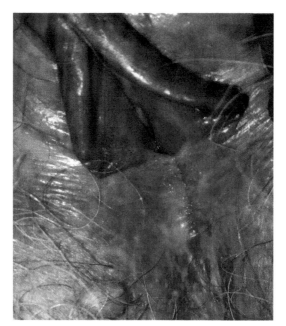

Fig. 1. Split at 6 o'clock on posterior fourchette in patient with lichen sclerosus.

Fissures Within Interlabial Sulci and Other Folds

These fissures can be due to infections, such as candida and herpes simplex, or due to inflammatory dermatoses, such as atopic dermatitis or lichen sclerosus. The cause also can be multifactorial; for example, due to candida superinfection in the context of atopic dermatitis or lichen sclerosus treated with topical corticosteroids.

Candida Infection Presentations
- Acute infection with marked pruritus and curdish, white vaginal discharge; splitting is not as pronounced
- Recurrent acute infections; clinical findings as in the previous bulleted item
- Chronic vulvovaginal candidiasis
  - Skin is dry
  - Minimal if any discharge
  - Splitting occurs in interlabial sulci and at the posterior fourchette
  - Lichenification can occur

All patients presenting with fissures should have swabs taken for microscopy and culture and testing for herpes simplex via polymerase chain reaction (PCR).

Fissures associated with the other causes listed occur in the presence of abnormal skin and mucous membrane surfaces of the vulva and generally occur within the natural creases and folds of vulvar tissue. Following the steps outlined previously should enable a diagnosis to be made and this will determine appropriate therapy.

Vulvar examination may not reveal fissures if the clinician does not gently but thoroughly examine all of the anogenital area, moving tissue such as the labia so that good visualization can be achieved.

Crohn disease of the vulva can cause long and deep fissures, knifelike linear ulcers with induration, in the absence of inflammatory bowel disease, and if not considered and a biopsy taken, the diagnosis will be missed.

Fissures due to pruritic dermatoses occur in areas of abnormal skin. Following the previously listed steps should enable a diagnosis to be made.

DRUG REACTIONS AFFECTING THE VULVA

The prevalence of drug eruptions has been reported to range from 2% to 5% for inpatients and more than 1% for outpatients in the United States.[3]

FIXED DRUG ERUPTION

Fixed drug eruption (FDE) is a reaction to a medication that once it has occurred will reoccur at the same site every time there is repeat exposure to the triggering agent. FDEs are thought to account for as much as 16% to 21% of all cutaneous drug eruptions. As many of the triggering agents (drugs, nutritional supplements) are readily available, the actual frequency may in fact be higher.[4]

The commonest clinical presentation is that of pigmented asymmetric erythematous circular/oval lesions that develop a central dusky erythematous area that can become bullous due to inflammation at the dermo-epidermal junction, resulting in an erosion if ruptured. Localized hyperpigmentation classically remains. Although it can occur anywhere on the skin, it does have a predilection for the orogenital skin.

Nonpigmenting FDE are more likely on the vulvar mucosa and this variant is more symmetric, erythematous, and plaquelike or erosive. Both variants recur at the same site with repeat exposure to the triggering drug.[5] Acute and chronic erosive vulvovaginitis has been reported as a presentation of nonpigmenting FDE due to nonsteroidal anti-inflammatory drugs (NSAIDs) and cholesterol-lowering agents.[6]

More recently, an eruption "generalized bullous FDE" has been described and distinguished by the authors from Stevens-Johnson syndrome (SJS)/toxic epidermal necrolysis (TEN).[7]

FDE occurs in response to medication taken orally, with antibiotics and NSAIDs being the most common culprits (**Box 4**). This box is by no means complete, with new culprits being reported often in the literature, but it does include the commonest groups of medications. The reactions generally occur within 30 minutes to 8 hours on initial exposure but can be delayed up to 48 hours, potentially complicating identifying the triggering agent.[8]

Box 4
Causes of fixed drug eruptions

- Pseudoephedrine
- Trimethoprim, sulfonamide (each on their own or in combination trimethoprim-sulfamethoxazole)
- Tetracycline
- Barbiturates
- Mefenamic acid
- Acetylsalicylic acid
- Phenolphthalein
- Ibuprofen
- Oxyphenbutazone
- Imidazoles

There have been reports in the literature in which vulvar FDE has been concluded to be oral medication taken by the sexual partners of these women and transferred in seminal fluid, adding another dimension of complexity to the history required to establish the culprit drug.[9]

In recent years, new techniques have enabled the identification of different populations of T cells, providing new insights into the pathogenesis of many drug reactions, including FDE. Memory T cells (TRM) that remain in lesional skin and react on reexposure to the triggering drugs occur on initial exposure and sensitization. The tissue localization of these cells is postulated to be why, despite Type IV hypersensitivity being the mechanism of reaction, patch testing is not useful unless it is done within the areas affected by the FDE.

TRMs also have been shown to provide long-lasting specific immunity to infection (eg, herpes virus) and are associated with recurring site-specific inflammatory diseases, such as cutaneous T-cell lymphoma.[10–12] An individual's susceptibility to FDE may be genetically determined in particular by HLA B22 status.[13]

Histopathological Findings

The biopsy must be taken at the edge of a lesion at the early eruptive stage for classic findings to be present. The changes are of an inflammatory dermatitis at the dermo-epidermal junction (interface dermatitis) with vacuolar changes. Civatte bodies (apoptotic basilar keratinocytes) are present. The location of the inflammatory infiltrate results in pigmentary incontinence, leaving the characteristic pigmentation seen in the classic variant of FDE.[14]

Lesions regress if the drug responsible is ceased after a plateau period of 3 to 5 days. The drugs that are known to trigger FDE are often common medications and include nutritional supplements that are available over-the-counter and may not be considered by patients as drugs. Nonpigmenting erosive genital FDE may resolve over a 2-week to 3-week time frame.

Investigations

- A careful history is the most useful diagnostic tool.
- Oral provocation tests with the suspected trigger drug have been used in the past to confirm a clinical suspicion, but as the eruptions can be severe, it is now not recommended.
- The current understanding of the pathogenic mechanism in FDE is that it is a Type IV hypersensitivity reaction involving sensitized T cells that remain in situ in affected tissue. Patch testing in the traditional location of the upper back has not proved helpful. Patch testing needs to be done in the location of the FDE, which in mucosal lesions is not practical.[15,16]

Management

The most important management point in these patients is to consider the differential diagnosis and identify and remove the triggering agent (see **Box 4**).

Class 1 (Super Potent) and Class 2 (Potent) corticosteroid ointments are generally sufficient to obtain resolution of localized FDE. Erosive nonpigmenting FDE presenting as erosive vulvovaginitis will usually respond to the same but intravaginal corticosteroid preparations, or short-course oral prednisolone may be necessary.

Avoidance of future exposure is essential, and patients should be given information on what to avoid, including cross-reacting triggers.

STEVENS-JOHNSON SYNDROME/TOXIC EPIDERMAL NECROSIS AND ERYTHEMA MULTIFORME MAJUS

SJS and TEN are currently considered opposite ends of a spectrum of severe epidermolytic drug reactions distinguished by the extent of epidermal loss. They have significant morbidity, and can be life-threatening, with mortality rates in TEN as high as 30%.[17] Drugs are considered responsible for 75% of SJS/TEN, with 25% being caused by mycoplasma pneumonia and other upper respiratory virus infections. Please note that the nomenclature can be confusing, as many people separate mycoplasma-induced presentations that are similar to SJS to be called mycoplasma-induced rash with mucositis rather than calling it SJS. They are very similar in terms of their clinical presentation as well as management. Erythema multiforme majus (EMM) has been determined to be a distinct unrelated condition[18–21] (**Table 2**).

The degree of epidermal loss or detachment is an important prognostic factor with the greater degree of loss associated with a poorer prognosis. Patients with SJS/TEN exhibit Nikolsky sign where the apparently attached epidermis can be loosened by gentle rubbing. Actual denuded areas and those exhibiting a positive Nikolsky sign should be included in determining the extent of epidermal involvement. Score for toxic epidermal necrosis (SCORTEN) is a validated system for determining disease severity and prognosis (**Tables 3** and **4**). Originally developed for TEN, it can and has been applied to other diseases involving epidermal necrosis.[22,23]

Pathogenesis

Although not completely and conclusively determined, the pathogenesis of SJS/TEN is currently considered an interplay of a patient's genetic susceptibility (HLAs), drug metabolism mechanisms, immunologic responses, T-cell clonotypes (CD 8+, natural killer cells) and cytokine changes. Ethnic predispositions appear to be the result of HLA associations and/or drug metabolism alterations, usually involving cytochrome p450 (**Table 5**).[18,24–26]

Histopathology

Timing of biopsies is important, as the most typical features are usually present at the beginning of lesion development and they should be taken at the earliest opportunity and from the edge of established lesions or, if possible, a lesion triggered by the Nikolsky sign.[27,28]

Early Erythematous Lesions
- Vacuolar change along the basement membrane zone, some lymphocytic infiltrate
- Civatte bodies; necrotic keratinocytes scattered throughout the inflammatory changes
- Variable, moderate perivascular and interstitial infiltrate in upper dermis, occasional eosinophils

Fully Developed/Later Lesion
- Subepithelial/subepidermal blistering or full-thickness epidermal/epithelial necrosis with apoptotic keratinocytes

Assessment and Management
- Presence of systemic symptoms
- Primary lesion(s) and their distribution

Table 2
Clinical features of SJS/TEN/EMM

DEMOGRAPHIC/ CLINICAL FEATURE	EMM	SJS	SJS/TEN	TEN
Patient age	<40 y	1–94 y, average 53 y		
Male:female ratio	M>F	1.0:1.1		
Systemic symptoms	Yes (100%)	1–94 y, average 53 y		
Primary lesions and distribution	Typical target lesions Mainly on limbs and palmar lesions Sometimes face and trunk	Dusky red lesions Atypical targets Individual lesions usually on face and trunk Epidermal detachment	Dusky red lesions starting to coalesce Atypical targets Increased epidermal detachment	Individual lesions less noticeable More extensive body involvement Increased epidermal detachment
Systemic symptoms	Yes	Usually	Yes	Yes
Epidermal loss	2%–5%	<10%	10%–30%	>30%
Mucosal involvement • Oral and ocular more common than genital • Erosive vulvovaginitis	100%	100%		
Etiology	Infections: (mainly) • Herpes simplex • Mycoplasma pneumoniae • Respiratory viruses Malignancy (usually blood) Drugs	Drugs: >75%–100% (more recent literature suggests the higher figure is more accurate, the other 25% representing other entities by current criteria) • Mycoplasma pneumoniae • Human immunodeficiency virus (HIV) infection affects T cells and increases risk of SJS/TEN due to sulfonamides		
"Incubation" period, d	3–14	4–28		
Pathogenetic differences	No autoantibodies against epithelial proteins (distinguishing finding)	• Genetically predisposed individuals (see **Table 5**) • Specific drugs have specific genetic predisposing factors • Drug-specific lesional lymphocyte-derived cytotoxic proteins causing epithelial destruction		

Abbreviations: EMM, erythema multiforme majus; SJS, Stevens-Johnson syndrome; TEN, toxic epidermal necrolysis.

Table 3
Score for toxic epidermal necrosis (SCORTEN)

Risk Factor	0	1
Age	<40 y	>40 y
Associated malignancy	No	Yes
Heart rate	<120	>120
Serum blood urea nitrogen, mg/dL	<28	>28
Degree of epidermal detachment	<10%	>10%
Serum bicarbonate, mEq/L	>20	<20
Serum glucose, mg/dL	<252	>252

The greater the score the worse the prognosis.

Table 4
Score for toxic epidermal necrosis (SCORTEN) (collation)

Number of Risk Factors	Mortality Rate, %
0–1	3.2
2	12.1
3	35.3
4	58.3
5 or more	>90.0

Table 5
Genetic/ethnic associations of Stevens-Johnson syndrome/toxic epidermal necrolysis

Drug	Genetic/Cytochrome p450 Association	Ethnic Group
Antibiotics		
Sulphonamides	HLA A 29, HLA B 12, HLA DR7	European
Sulfamethoxazole	HLA B 38	European
Anticonvulsants		
Carbamazepine	HLA B 15:02	Han Chinese, Thai, Indian, Malaysian
	HLA B15:11	Japanese, Korean, Han Chinese
	HLA B 59:01	Japanese
	HLA A 31:01	Japanese, north European
Lamotegrine	HLA B 15:02	Han Chinese
Oxcarbazepine	HLA B 15:02	Han Chinese
Phenytoin	HLA B 15:02	Han Chinese
	CYP2C93	Han Chinese, Japanese, Malaysian
Nonsteroidal anti-inflammatory drugs		
Oxicam	HLA A 2, HLA B 12 HLA B 73	European
Antiretrovirals		
Nevirapine	CYP2B6 HLA C 04:01	African (Mozambique) African (Malawi)
Xanthine oxidase inhibitors		
Allopurinol	HLA B 58:01	Han Chinese, Thai, Japanese, Korean, European

- Extent of epidermal loss
- History of possible infective triggers over the past 8 weeks
- History of medications: prescribed, self-administered including nutritional supplements (also over the past 8 weeks)
- Biopsy
- Blood tests to determine disease severity, human immunodeficiency virus (HIV) status (see **Tables 4** and **5**)
- Adjunctive genetic studies, if available, to establish if a patient has an HLA or cytochrome p450 identity known to be associated with SJS/TEN (**Table 6**)
- General medical history to help determine possible underlying internal disorders
- Determine the overall disease severity (SCORTEN)
- Determine likely drug causality: Algorithm of Drug Causality for Epidermal Necrolysis (ALDEN): an algorithm for the assessment of drug causality in SJS/TEN, developed by the RegiSCAR Study Group[29]

Treatment

There is no consensus on the therapy of SJS/TEN or EMM. Treatment is generally symptomatic and supportive determined by disease extent and severity[30]:

- Identification and withdrawal of the suspected causative drug or treatment of causative infection
- Admission into appropriate unit where general supportive care can be given; for example, burns unit, intensive care unit
- Referral to colleagues to implement specific treatment of involved systems; for example, ophthalmologists, gastroenterologists, surgeons
- Systemic therapy may be used, such as intravenous immunoglobulins, cyclosporine, high-dose oral glucocorticoids, tumor necrosis factor (TNF)-α inhibitors[31]

Genitourinary care

As with nonmucosal disease, there is no consensus on the management of genitourinary involvement in the SJS/TEN continuum. Unfortunately, mucosal lesions do not respond as well to immunomodulation, and there are well-documented long-standing sequelae for which prevention is still a therapeutic challenge.[32,33] The anogenital region should be examined in all women admitted to hospital, as involvement may not

Table 6
Recommended treatment options for first clinical episode of genital herpes simplex virus

Drug and Dose	Frequency, Times per d	Duration, d
Acyclovir, 400 mg	3	7–10
Acyclovir, 200 mg	5	7–10
Famciclovir 250 mg	3	7–10
Valacyclovir 1 g	2	7–10

Treatment can be extended if complete healing has not occurred.

It is suggested that readers access the Centers for Disease Control and Prevention Web site for the most up-to-date recommendations within United States and their corresponding regulatory bodies in other parts of the world.

Adapted from Centers for Disease Control and Prevention (CDC). 2015 sexually transmitted diseases treatment guidelines: genital HSV infections. Available at: http://www.cdc.gov/std/tg2015/herpes.htm. Accessed August 25, 2016.

be the major problem initially but can occur later. The following are the principles of vulvovaginal care and treatment in SJS/TEN:

- Pain relief
- Prevention of secondary infection
- Prevention of urinary retention
- Prevention of adhesions: urethral and vaginal introital stenosis
- Long-term follow-up if involved looking to manage scarring, possible development of vaginal adenosis, dyspareunia, apareunia

Therapeutic interventions include the following:
- Urinary catheterization
- Sitz baths or regular cleansing in an ill and immobile patient with application of nonadherent or wet dressings if practical
- The insertion of tampons or vaginal dilators covered with emollients, such as paraffin or petrolatum, and replaced twice a day or daily
- Potent or super-potent corticosteroid preparations, such as betamethasone dipropionate also can be used in severe cases, although mild topical corticosteroid ointments can be soothing
- Vaginal application with a latex-free dilator is possibly preferable to a tampon in extensive vaginal involvement to ensure greater vaginal coverage and to maintain patency, as well as to lower infectious risk with the use of a tampon
- Ointment bases are preferred, as they contain less preservative and provide superior barrier protection
- The use of antifungal creams to prevent supervening candidiasis has been proposed. These can be irritating, and consideration should be given to the use of oral agents
- Vaginal molds for use during the acute phase and until complete healing has occurred also have been suggested. As with dilators, these can be combined with the use of topical corticosteroids
- Menstrual suppression in women of reproductive age
- The previously listed intravaginal devices are not recommended in the pediatric population

Special Considerations in Pregnant Women
- Monitoring of fetal status for possible fetal stress.
- Review delivery methods if appropriate. Both vaginal and cesarean deliveries have been used as determined by the general health of the mother and the degree of vulvovaginal involvement at time of delivery. Examination for possible introital stenosis and vaginal synechiae are indicated in women who have healed from SJS/TEN.
- Maternal and fetal involvement in SJS/TEN in the acute phase: fetal involvement simultaneously with maternal has been reported with the possibility of fetal death.[34] Most deliveries reported in the literature have been of healthy babies.
- HIV status determination. HIV infection increases the risk of SJS/TEN substantially in pregnancy, particularly in women receiving retroviral therapy with nevirapine.[35,36]

HERPES SIMPLEX INFECTION: HERPES VIRUS 1 AND 2, VARICELLA ZOSTER VIRUS

Herpes simplex virus (HSV) is the commonest cause of vulvar erosions/ulcers. Both HSV 1 and 2 cause herpes simplex genitalis (HSG). Traditionally, HSV1 has been predominantly responsible for herpes simplex labialis and HSV 2, HSG. Varicella zoster virus (VZV) is another herpes virus than can affect the genitalia, although less commonly. Current treatment regimens with antiviral drugs are outlined in **Tables 6–8**.

These herpes viruses are double-stranded DNA viruses classified as members of the alpha Herpesviridae family. They share the following characteristics:

- Infections are lifelong infections once acquired
- They remain latent in the sensory ganglia associated with the primary infection
- The skin and mucous membranes are the path of entry into the body
- Vertical transmission can occur from mother to infant during vaginal delivery
- Clinically, HSV1 and HSV2 cannot be distinguished
- Most genital herpes infections are sexually acquired
- HSV infections and FDE are the 2 clinical entities that recur in the same spot on the skin or mucous membranes

Epidemiology

Serologic population studies are the most effective epidemiologic tool in HSV infections. In the United States, nearly 1 in 5 adults (approximately 50 million persons) has HSV2 infection, with 1 million new infections occurring each year.[37,38]

HSV1 is becoming increasingly acquired genitally and now represents at least half of new infections. This is thought to reflect changes in sexual practices with an increase in orogenital sex.[39]

The true prevalence of undiagnosed HSV2 is unknown, but serologic screening suggests many primary infections are asymptomatic. The seroprevalence in the United States between 2005 and 2010 was 16%, but only 14% of seropositive individuals reported a history of HSG. Viral shedding from asymptomatic individuals occurs in a substantial number of infected individuals. Most presentations of HSG are likely to be reactivation of latent HSV infections.[40] The severity and frequency of the disease and the recurrence rate depend on numerous factors, including viral type, prior immunity to autologous or heterologous virus, gender, and immune status of the host.

Table 7
Episodic treatment for recurrent herpes simplex genitalis

Drug and Dose	Frequency	Duration, d
Acyclovir, 400 mg	Three times a day	5
Acyclovir, 800 mg	Twice a day	5
Acyclovir, 800 mg	Three times a day	2
Famciclovir 125 mg	Twice a day	5
Famciclovir, 1 g	Twice a day	1
Famciclovir, 500 mg and 250 mg	Single dose of 500 mg on day 1, followed by 250 mg twice per day on days 2 and 3	3
Valacyclovir 500 mg	Twice a day	3
Valacyclovir, 1 g	Daily	5

It is suggested that readers access the Centers for Disease Control and Prevention Web site for the most up-to-date recommendations within the United States and their corresponding regulatory bodies in other parts of the world.

Adapted from Centers for Disease Control and Prevention (CDC). 2015 sexually transmitted diseases treatment guidelines: genital HSV infections. Available at: http://www.cdc.gov/std/tg2015/herpes.htm. Accessed August 25, 2016.

Table 8	
Suppressive therapy for recurrent herpes simplex genitalis	
Drug and Dose	Frequency, Times per d
Acyclovir, 400 mg	2
Famciclovir	2
Valacyclovir 500 mg	2
Valacyclovir 1 g	1

It is suggested that readers access the Centers for Disease Control and Prevention Web site for the most up-to-date recommendations within the United States and their corresponding regulatory bodies in other parts of the world.

Adapted from Centers for Disease Control and Prevention (CDC). 2015 sexually transmitted diseases treatment guidelines: genital HSV infections. Available at: http://www.cdc.gov/std/tg2015/herpes.htm. Accessed August 25, 2016.

Primary Herpes Simplex Genitalis

Cause
- HSV1 and 2. The viruses are present in saliva; urine; vulvar, vaginal, and cervical secretions; and in seminal fluid. Close contact is required for spread.[41]

Incubation period
- 3 to 7 days (1 day to 3 weeks)

Clinical Features
- Constitutional: fever, malaise, headache, myalgia.
- Local: pain, itching, dysuria, vaginal discharge, edema.
- Regional: tenderness and aching in the inguinal areas due to lymphadenopathy.
- Vulvar lesions: patient may report small, tender bumps on the vulva initially, although these quickly rupture and tenderness and pain may be the only symptoms.
- Duration: 14 days to heal the erosions.
- Virus travels along axon to sensory ganglion of corresponding spinal level during the infective stage and remains there, latent, for life.

Examination findings:
- Herpetic lesions can occur anywhere in the anogenital area, including the vagina and cervix. Vesicles may be seen, but as the viral damage is intraepithelial, they will quickly denude, leaving exquisitely tender erosions, occasionally ulcers. Urethritis may be present, but dysuria also can be the result of urine contacting denuded vulvar tissue.
- Difficulty with micturition can occur as a consequence of these factors as well as edema. Urinary retention may occur, requiring catheterization.
- Vaginitis is usually erosive and edematous. Cervical involvement has been estimated at 70% to 90%; however, a speculum examination is not recommended as part of the initial examination because of pain and the possibility of introducing secondary infection.

Investigations
- Tzanck smear can be done by the bedside looking for multinucleated giant cells in tissue/exudate scraped from the blister base.
- PCR or direct fluorescent antibody testing from vesicular fluid, if present, or base of newest lesion. False negatives increase dramatically after first 24 to 48 hours.

Risk factors
- Sexual activity with a partner who is shedding virus (active lesions, immunocompromised).
- Immunocompromised individual.
- Broken skin: preexisting dermatosis; atopic eczema, vigorous sexual activity.
- Atopic eczema (increased susceptibility to herpetic infections).

Recurrent Herpes Simplex Genitalis

These are the usual clinical presentations seen by clinicians, and a history of a severe primary episode, as detailed previously, is not always present. Eighty percent of primary infections are asymptomatic. Reactivation of HSG causes migration of the HSV along the infected and contralateral axons to the skin and mucous membranes. In women, lesions can occur anywhere in the anogenital region, with vesicles, when noted, tending to occur in areas, such as the labia majora or perineum, that have thicker epithelium.

Recurrent episodes are overall shorter in duration and may lack a constitutional prodrome.[42] A pronounced prodrome should raise the suspicion that the individual is immunocompromised. The presenting history is more likely to be dominated by localized vulvar symptoms of pruritus, paresthesia, or vulvar "bumps," but usually a recurrent tender spot or fissure, occurring in the same area on each occasion. In some patients, severe ipsilateral sacral neuralgia occurs[43] (**Fig. 2**).

The natural history of HSG is that recurrences become less severe and less common over time. Facial and oral HSV1 infection results in the production of antibodies that offer protection from HSG due to this virus but not protection from infection with HSV2. Interestingly, the presence of these antibodies is thought to reduce the severity of HSV2 infections. The lesions heal in 8 to 10 days, and viral shedding lasts an average 5 days. The symptoms are more severe in women than men.

Herpes Simplex Genitalis in Immunocompromised Women

Immunocompetence can be the result of a variety of factors. As a predominantly sexually acquired infection, HSG influences the risk of an individual acquiring other sexually transmitted infections either simultaneously or during recurrent episodes when the normal barrier function of the vulvar tissue is compromised.

Specific history to determine immunocompetency
- General health: adequate nutrition
- Solid organ or bone marrow transplantation
- Medications for treatment of arthritis; skin disease, for example, psoriasis; inflammatory bowel disease
  - Methotrexate
  - TNF-α inhibitors
- Bone marrow dyscrasias: myelodysplasia, chronic lymphocytic leukemia (**Fig. 3**)
- HIV infections (may be undiagnosed)
- A past history of HSG may be absent
- HSV2 positivity increases the risk of HIV acquisition in at-risk individuals[44]
- The infectiveness of both HIV and HSV2 increases during recurrences of HSG in HIV-positive individuals[45]
- Suppressive HSV antiviral therapy reduces genital and plasma HIV levels in women with concurrent HSG/HIV infection[46]

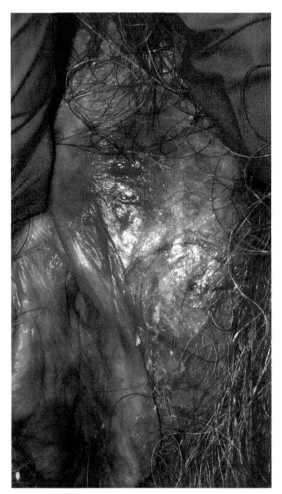

Fig. 2. Recurrent HSG in a patient with lichen sclerosus using potent topical corticosteroids.

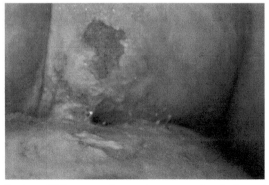

Fig. 3. Extension of vulvar HSG over perineum to anus and onto inner buttocks in patient immunosuppressed due to having chronic lymphocytic leukemia. (*Courtesy of* D. Dyall-Smith, MBBS, FACD, Wagga Wagga, New South Wales, Australia.)

Differences in presentation of HSG in immunocompromised patients
- The presentation may be more severe and prolonged
- A clinical prodrome more reminiscent of a primary episode may be present along with atypical clinical features, progression, and a poor response to therapy
- Lesions can become deeper and more expansive, extending beyond the vulva to involve the perianal area, buttocks, and inner thighs
- Progression is by direct extension, with increased depth and possibly eschar formation
- Swabs for HSV PCR may be negative, and biopsy of the extending edge is often useful
- Secondary infection has to be continuously searched for and treated accordingly
- Surgical debridement and grafting may be required, but should not be attempted before total control of the infection is achieved
- Management of the immunosuppression should be reviewed. This may be able to be modified to aid control of the infection and prevent recurrences that are more likely in these women. When this is not possible, long-term continuous antiviral therapy is needed.

Herpes Simplex Genitalis Investigations and Therapy

- PCR assay is the preferred test for confirming HSV in clinically apparent lesions
- Suppressive therapy reduces symptom severity, duration, and recurrence in patients with HSG
- In HIV-negative patients, suppressive therapy is effective in reducing transmission to at-risk partners
- In persons with HIV and HSV2 infections, suppressive therapy does not reduce the transmission of HSV to at-risk partners
- Serology for HSV is not recommended as a diagnostic investigation, but may be considered in partners to guide counseling
- Length of antiviral therapy at therapeutic doses should be until lesions are fully healed, which is often longer than a typical course and may take weeks to more than a month
- If diagnosis is confirmed but the patient is not responding to usual HSV treatment, consider acyclovir resistance or cytomegalovirus coinfection

Complications of Herpes Simplex Genitalis More Common in Immunocompromised Individuals

- Aseptic meningitis (including a recurrent form)
- Disseminated herpes
- Encephalitis
- Hepatitis
- Neonatal infection
- Pelvic inflammatory disease
- Pneumonitis

There are no recommended regimens for antiviral drug therapy in immunocompromised patients. The dose should be adjusted upward until control and subsequent healing occurs. Suppressive therapy is more appropriate in this group of patients than episodic therapy.

Varicella Zoster Virus Infection

- The clinical presentation of localized varicella zoster virus (VZV) or "shingles" is characteristically a pustule-vesicular eruption confined to one dermatome. The

pathognomonic clinical feature is the involvement of one side of the vulva only, with lesions not crossing the midline.
- Contiguous dermatomes may be involved, but spread should not extend further in the immunocompetent woman. The lesions are intraepithelial and therefore form erosions rather than ulcers and are painful.
- Superinfection can occur.
- Rarely, herpes simplex virus (HSV) can occur in a dermatomal distribution and mimic HZV. The diagnosis is usually a clinical one, but PCR testing of a swab taken from vesicular fluid or the base of a lesion within the first 48 hours of eruption will confirm diagnosis.
- Reactivation of herpes varicella zoster should always signal the clinician to assess the general health of the patient. Blood and bone marrow disorders, in particular, should be excluded.
- Extension beyond contiguous dermatomes or disseminated spread of lesions, which are typical of chicken pox, should alert the clinician to an underlying cause of immune-impairment.
- Disseminated varicella is associated with potential severe systemic end-organ compromise and even death; thus, it warrants hospitalization, careful monitoring, and aggressive antiviral treatment.

Treatment options are based on the following:
- Patient age
- Patient immune state
- Duration of symptoms
- Presentation

High-risk patients
- Pregnant women
- Immunocompromised women
- Adults without evidence of immunity

Acyclovir resistance is sometimes seen. The drugs and doses for VZV of the vulva are the same as those for primary HSG.

SUMMARY

A knowledge of normal vulvar anatomy, a thorough history, and a careful physical examination are the foundation to evaluating patients with vulvar fissures and erosions. These tools will help formulate a differential diagnosis that will direct further investigation to eventually establish a working diagnosis and appropriate treatment plan. Clinicians must be prepared to revisit their evaluation and assessment if patient progress is not as expected.

REFERENCES

1. The Australian STI Management Guidelines. Available at: http://www.sexualhealthalliance.org.au/ASHA. Accessed April 2016.
2. Barbero M, Micheletti L, Valentino MC, et al. Membranous hypertrophy of the posterior fourchette as a cause of dyspareunia and vulvodynia. J Reprod Med 1994; 39(12):949–52.
3. Krahenbuhl-Melcher A, Schlienger R, Lampert M, et al. Drug-related problems in hospitals: a review of the recent literature. Drug Saf 2007;30(5):379–407.
4. Lee AY. Fixed drug eruptions. Incidence, recognition, and avoidance. Am J Clin Dermatol 2000;1(5):277–85.

5. Shelley WB, Shelley D. Nonpigmenting fixed drug eruption as a distinctive reaction pattern: examples caused by sensitivity to pseudoephedrine hydrochloride and tetrahydrozoline. J Am Acad Dermatol 1987;17(3):403–7.

6. Fischer G. Vulvar fixed drug eruption. A report of 13 cases. J Reprod Med 2007; 52(2):81–6.

7. Lipowicz S, Sekula P, Ingen-Housz-Oro S, et al. Prognosis of generalized bullous fixed drug eruption: comparison with Stevens-Johnson syndrome and toxic epidermal necrolysis. Br J Dermatol 2013;168(4):726–32.

8. Korkij W, Soltani K. Fixed drug eruption. A brief review. Arch Dermatol 1984; 120(4):520–4.

9. Zawar V, Chuh A. Fixed drug eruption may be sexually induced. Int J Dermatol 2006;45:1003–4.

10. Park CO, Kupper TS. The emerging role of resident memory T cells in protective immunity and inflammatory disease. Nat Med 2015;21(7):688–97.

11. Mizukawa Y, Yamazaki Y, Shiohara T. In vivo dynamics of intraepidermal CD8+ Tcells and CD4+ Tcells during the evolution of fixed drug eruption. Br J Dermatol 2008;158(6):1230–8.

12. Mizukawa Y, Shiohara T. Fixed drug eruption: a prototypic disorder mediated by effector memory T cells. Curr Allergy Asthma Rep 2009;9(1):71–7.

13. Pellicano R, Ciavarella G, Lomuto M, et al. Genetic susceptibility to fixed drug eruption: evidence for a link with HLA-B22. J Am Acad Dermatol 1994;30(1):52–4.

14. Weedon D. The lichenoid reaction pattern ('interface dermatitis'). In: Weedon D, editor. Skin pathology. 2nd edition. London: Churchill Livingstone; 2002. p. 42–3.

15. Shiohara T. Fixed drug eruption: pathogenesis and diagnostic tests. Curr Opin Allergy Clin Immunol 2009;9(4):316–21.

16. Mizukawa Y, Yamazaki Y, Teraki Y, et al. Direct evidence for interferon-gamma production by effector-memory-type in intraepidermal T cells residing at an effector site of immunopathology in fixed drug eruption. Am J Pathol 2002; 161(4):1337–47.

17. Knowles S, Shear NH. Clinical risk management of Stevens-Johnson syndrome/ toxic epidermal necrolysis spectrum. Dermatol Ther 2009;22(5):441–51.

18. Dodiuk-Gad RP, Chung W-H, Valeyrie-Allanore L, et al. Stevens–Johnson syndrome and toxic epidermal necrolysis: an update. Am J Clin Dermatol 2015; 16(6):475–93.

19. Mockenhaupt M. The current understanding of Stevens–Johnson syndrome and toxic epidermal necrolysis. Expert Rev Clin Immunol 2011;7(6):803–13.

20. Schwartz RA, McDonough PH, Lee BW. Toxic epidermal necrolysis: part I. Introduction, history, classification, clinical features, systemic manifestations, etiology, and immunopathogenesis. J Am Acad Dermatol 2013;69(2):173.e1-13.

21. Auquier-Dunant A, Mockenhaupt M, Naldi L, et al. Correlations between clinical patterns and causes of erythema multiforme majus, Stevens–Johnson syndrome, and toxic epidermal necrolysis: results of an international prospective study. Arch Dermatol 2002;138(8):1019–24.

22. Bastuji-Garin S, Fouchard N, Bertocchi M, et al. SCORTEN: a severity-of-illness score for toxic epidermal necrolysis. J Invest Dermatol 2000;115(2):149–53.

23. Sekula P, Liss Y, Davidovici B, et al. Evaluation of SCORTEN on a cohort of patients with Stevens–Johnson syndrome and toxic epidermal necrolysis included in the RegiSCAR study. J Burn Care Res 2011;32(2):237–45.

24. Alfirevic A, Pirmohamed M. Drug induced hypersensitivity and the HLA complex. Pharmaceuticals 2011;4:69–90.

25. Hershfield MS, Callaghan JT, Tassaneeyakul W, et al. Clinical Pharmacogenetics Implementation Consortium guidelines for human leukocyte antigen-B genotype and allopurinol dosing. Clin Pharmacol Ther 2013;93(2):153–8.

26. Genin E, Chen DP, Hung SI, et al. HLA-A*31:01 and different types of carbamazepine-induced severe cutaneous adverse reactions: an international study and meta-analysis. Pharmacogenomics J 2014;14(3):281–8.

27. Valeyrie-Allanore L, Bastuji-Garin S, Guegan S, et al. Prognostic value of histologic features of toxic epidermal necrolysis. J Am Acad Dermatol 2013;68(2):e29–35.

28. Quinn AM, Brown K, Bonish BK, et al. Uncovering histologic criteria with prognostic significance in toxic epidermal necrolysis. Arch Dermatol 2005;141(6): 683–7.

29. Sassolas B, Haddad C, Mockenhaupt M, et al. ALDEN, an algorithm for assessment of drug causality in Stevens–Johnson syndrome and toxic epidermal necrolysis: comparison with case–control analysis. Clin Pharmacol Ther 2010;88(1): 60–8.

30. Fromowitz JS, Ramos-Caro FA, Flowers FP, et al. Practical guidelines for the management of toxic epidermal necrolysis and Stevens–Johnson syndrome. Int J Dermatol 2007;46(10):1092–4.

31. Abela C, Hartmann CE, De Leo A, et al. Toxic epidermal necrolysis (TEN): the Chelsea and Westminster Hospital wound management algorithm. J Plast Reconstr Aesthet Surg 2014;67(8):1026–32.

32. Kaser DJ, Reichman DE, Laufer MR. Prevention of vulvovaginal sequelae in Stevens–Johnson syndrome and toxic epidermal necrolysis. Rev Obstet Gynecol 2011;4(2):81–5.

33. Niemeijer IC, van Praag MC, van Gemund N. Relevance and consequences of erythema multiforme, Stevens–Johnson syndrome and toxic epidermal necrolysis in gynecology. Arch Gynecol Obstet 2009;280(5):851–4.

34. Struck MF, Illert T, Liss Y, et al. Toxic epidermal necrolysis in pregnancy: case report and review of the literature. J Burn Care Res 2010;31(5):816–21.

35. Dube N, Adewusi E, Summers R. Risk of nevirapine-associated Stevens–Johnson syndrome among HIV-infected pregnant women: the Medunsa National Pharmacovigilance Centre, 2007–2012. S Afr Med J 2013;103(5):322–5.

36. Knight L, Muloiwa R, Dlamini S, et al. Factors associated with increased mortality in a predominantly HIV-infected population with Stevens Johnson syndrome and toxic epidermal necrolysis. PLoS One 2014;9(4):e93543.

37. Bernstein DI, Bellamy AR, Hook EW III, et al. Epidemiology, clinical presentation, and antibody response to primary infection with herpes simplex virus type 1 and type 2 in young women. Clin Infect Dis 2013;56(3):344–51.

38. Centers for Disease Control and Prevention (CDC). Seroprevalence of herpes simplex virus type 2 among persons aged 14-49 years—United States, 2005-2008. MMWR Morb Mortal Wkly Rep 2010;59(15):456–9.

39. Bradley H, Markowitz LE, Gibson T, et al. Seroprevalence of herpes simplex virus types 1 and 2—United States, 1999-2010. J Infect Dis 2014;209(3):325–33.

40. Tronstein E, Johnston C, Huang ML, et al. Genital shedding of herpes simplex virus among symptomatic and asymptomatic persons with HSV-2 infection. JAMA 2011;305(14):1441–9.

41. Kimberlin DW, Rouse DJ. Clinical practice. Genital herpes. N Engl J Med 2004; 350(19):1970–7.

42. Benedetti JK, Zeh J, Corey L. Clinical reactivation of genital herpes simplex virus infection decreases in frequency over time. Ann Intern Med 1999;131(1):14–20.

43. Freeman EE, Weiss HA, Glynn JR, et al. Herpes simplex virus 2 infection increases HIV acquisition in men and women: systematic review and meta-analysis of longitudinal studies. AIDS 2006;20(1):73–83.

44. Gupta R, Warren T, Wald A. Genital herpes. Lancet 2007;370(9605):2127–37.

45. Corey L, Wald A, Celum CL, et al. The effects of herpes simplex virus-2 on HIV-1 acquisition and transmission: a review of two overlapping epidemics. J Acquir Immune Defic Syndr 2004;35(5):435–45.

46. Baeten JM, Strick LB, Lucchetti A, et al. Herpes simplex virus (HSV)-suppressive therapy decreases plasma and genital HIV-1 levels in HSV-2/HIV-1 coinfected women: a randomized, placebo-controlled, cross-over trial. J Infect Dis 2008; 198(12):1804–8.

A Clinical Approach to Vulvar Ulcers

Kristen M.A. Stewart, MD

KEYWORDS

- Vulvar • Ulcer • Differential diagnosis • Treatment

KEY POINTS

- Vulvar ulcers are nonspecific skin findings.
- The differential diagnosis of vulvar ulcers is broad.
- Vulvar ulcers are frequently misdiagnosed on clinical examination.
- Laboratory testing is usually required for accurate diagnosis.

VULVAR ULCERS

Background

Most vulvar ulcers are painful and trigger considerable anxiety and emotional distress for the patient. Any form of vulvar irritation or discomfort affects all aspects of a patient's life, including simple activities of daily living, exercise, and sexual encounters. In addition to physical pain and discomfort, however, there are also often underlying fears that the symptoms are due to a sexually transmitted infection, undiagnosed cancer, poor hygiene, or that there will never be relief,[1] leading to psychological effects on the well-being of relationships and the patient's feelings of self-worth.

Providers are often challenged to determine the cause of this nonspecific clinical sign and institute appropriate therapy. Ulcerative vulvar conditions include a spectrum of primary examination findings, including ulcers, erosions, and other ulcerated lesions, such as sinus tracts and draining nodules. This article seeks to provide a practical clinical approach to the evaluation of ulcerative vulvar disease.

Ulcers of the vulva are diagnostically challenging due to variation in clinical morphology. Accurately identifying the primary morphology is clinically relevant because most disease states produce either erosions or ulcerations, and correctly identifying the primary lesion can significantly narrow the differential diagnosis.[2] Determining the primary morphology of a vulvar ulcer, however, is often complicated by secondary changes and that more than a single condition is often present.

There are no financial disclosures or conflicts of interest to report.
Total Dermatology Care Center P.A., 915 West Monroe Street, Suite 101, Jacksonville, FL 32204, USA
E-mail address: kstewart@totaldermcare.com

Obstet Gynecol Clin N Am 44 (2017) 445–451
http://dx.doi.org/10.1016/j.ogc.2017.05.010
0889-8545/17/© 2017 Elsevier Inc. All rights reserved.

obgyn.theclinics.com

Vulvar ulcers are a symptom, and an underlying cause must not be assumed but rather must be sought. Diagnosis based solely on clinical findings is often inaccurate. Identifying the cause of a vulvar ulcer is best accomplished by obtaining a careful history, performing a detailed physical examination, and considering a broad differential diagnosis. Although the most common causes of vulvar ulcers are sexually transmitted infections, it is imperative to maintain a broad approach by considering the range of nonsexually transmitted causes.[3] A study of 53 women presenting for evaluation of genital ulcers at a clinic in Brazil, for example, showed that 54.7% of cases were associated with sexually transmitted infections and that the remaining 45.3% of cases resulted from other causes.[4] The differential diagnosis includes sexually and nonsexually transmitted infections, dermatoses, trauma, neoplasms, hormonally induced ulcers, and drug reactions (**Box 1**).

Patient History

Using a patient questionnaire tailored to your practice can facilitate and expedite the patient encounter (**Box 2**). The interview should start with the patient's defining her symptoms. This definition may be facilitated by offering a variety of descriptors, such as burn, rawness, pain, tingling, irritation, and itch. Next, define the location (unifocal, multiple areas, or generalized) and onset (chronicity, recurrence) of the symptoms, as well as any potentially relevant circumstances.

Review in detail the signs and symptoms at onset and their evolution over time. Ask the patient to identify potential triggers, anything that makes the symptoms better or worse, and previous similar eruptions. Clarify management before presentation, including over-the-counter (OTC) treatments, home remedies, and prescriptions; determine the length of use and the results of such treatments. Inquire about personal hygiene routines and products, including cleansers, douches, use of washcloths and wet wipes, sanitary pads, and tampons. Determine how the products are used and how frequently. Review the patient's sexual experience and travel history, including gender of sexual contacts; new, anonymous, or high-risk partners; number of sexual contacts in last month and last 6 months; geographic locations of sexual contacts; anatomical sites of sexual contacts; history of previous sexually transmitted infections; and use of barrier protection.

Gather pertinent past medical history, including allergies; OTC and prescription medications, with emphasis on any changes in the 6 months before symptom onset; immune status; systemic disease; relevant surgeries; age of menarche; and last menstrual period. Conduct a directed review of systems, including fever, fatigue, headache, muscle pain, nausea, vomiting, anorexia, abdominal pain, skin eruption or rash, oral lesions, pain with swallowing, vaginal discharge, pain with intercourse, pain with urination, cold or flu-like symptoms, eye irritation, blurred vision, depression, and anxiety. Identify any pertinent family history of genital ulcers, Behçet disease, Crohn disease, and lupus or other autoimmune disease.

Physical Examination

The physical examination should include a whole-body mucocutaneous examination, focusing on the skin, eyes, oropharynx, anogenital areas, lymph nodes, and joints. Because vaginal disease can have great effect on the vulva, the vaginal mucosa should be included in the examination. A sample of the vaginal secretions should be studied microscopically for the presence of clue cells, lactobacilli, hyphae, pseudohyphae, or budding yeast. Inspect the entire vulva for ulcers, erosions, fissures, subtle erythema, friability, induration, edema, lichenification, crusting, atrophy, and hyperpigmentation or hypopigmentation, as well as the presence of scarring and

Box 1
Differential diagnosis of vulvar ulcers

Infectious

Sexually transmitted
  Herpes simplex virus
  Syphilis
  Chancroid
  Granuloma inguinale
  Lymphogranuloma venereum
  Human immunodeficiency virus

Nonsexually transmitted
  Epstein-Barr virus
  Herpes zoster (varicella-zoster virus)
  Cytomegalovirus
  Hand, foot, and mouth disease
  Candidiasis
  Bacterial infections (staphylococcus, streptococcus, *Mycoplasma pneumoniae*)

Noninfectious

Dermatitides
  Nonbullous
    Hidradenitis suppurativa
    Crohn disease
    Aphthous ulcers
    Behçet disease
    Contact dermatitis (allergic or irritant contact)
    Lupus erythematosus
    Pyoderma gangrenosum
    Graft-versus-host disease
    Lichen planus
    Lichen sclerosus
    Zoon vulvitis
  Bullous
    Bullous pemphigoid
    Cicatricial pemphigoid
    Pemphigus vulgaris
    Linear immunoglobulin A disease
    Hailey-Hailey disease
    Epidermolysis bullosa acquisita

Trauma
  Blunt, sharp
  Heat, cold
  Factitial
  Female genital mutilation

Neoplasms
  Basal cell carcinoma
  Squamous cell carcinoma
  Vulvar intraepithelial neoplasia
  Extramammary Paget disease
  Verrucous carcinoma
  Melanoma
  Lymphoma
  Leukemia
  Hodgkin disease

Hormonally induced
  Autoimmune progesterone dermatitis
  Estrogen hypersensitivity

Drug reactions
  Fixed drug eruption
  Toxic epidermal necrolysis
  Erythema multiforme

Box 2
Information to obtain from patient

Age, allergies, past medical history, past surgical history.

List over-the-counter and prescription (Rx) medications, as well as herbal and dietary supplements, that you take daily.

List OTC and Rx medications, as well as herbal and dietary supplements, that you take as needed only.

List OTC and Rx medications, as well as herbal and dietary supplements, that were started in the last 6 months.

List all products and treatments (OTC and Rx) that come into contact with your genital skin, including cleansers, soap, washcloth, powders, moisturizers, sprays, wet wipes, creams, ointments, and so forth.

Describe your discomfort: itch, rawness, soreness, burning, or other.

When did your symptoms start?

Can you think of anything that might have triggered your symptoms?

Do any specific triggers make the symptoms worse, such as sexual activity, menstrual period, exercise, or treatment? Does anything make the symptoms better?

Have you noticed any change in vaginal discharge?

What have you tried to treat your symptoms?

Have you ever had similar symptoms in the past? When? Treatment?

When was your last menstrual period? Menopause at what age?

What sanitary products do you use during you menstrual period: panty liners, pads, tampons, scented versus unscented?

Do you use any hormonal replacement: oral, transdermal patch, intravaginal (cream, ring, suppository)?

Are you sexually active?
  Do you have sex with men? Women? Both?
  Do you have oral sexual contact? Vulvovaginal? Anal?
  Do you use any lubrication products? What products?
  Do you use any contraception? What type?
  Do you use condoms? How often?
  Have you had a new, anonymous, or high-risk sex partner?
  Number of sexual contacts in last month? Last 6 months?
  Have you, or your sexual partners, traveled outside the United States? Where?

Have you ever been told that you have or had any of the following: an abnormal pap smear, genital warts, herpes, shingles, gonorrhea, chlamydia, hepatitis, syphilis, HIV?

Are you currently experiencing any of the following: fever, fatigue, headache, muscle pain, nausea, vomiting, anorexia, abdominal pain, skin eruption or rash, oral lesions, pain with swallowing, vaginal discharge, pain with intercourse, pain with urination, cold or flu-like symptoms, eye irritation, blurred vision, depression, or anxiety?

Does anyone in your family have a history of any of the following: genital ulcers, Behçet disease, Crohn disease, lupus, or other autoimmune disease?

loss of architecture. Document the number, type, size, border characteristics, depth, type of exudate if present, location, tenderness, and description of primary lesions, as well as the presence or absence of local lymphadenopathy and any extragenital findings.

It can be difficult to ascertain the morphology of the primary lesion and specifically to resolve whether the primary lesion is an ulcer or an erosion. Erosions involve loss of the epidermis only and often appear as deep red macules or patches. Ulcers are deeper than erosions and characterized by loss of both epidermis and dermis. On examination, an ulcer typically appears with a white or yellowish fibrinous base. Erosions can be transformed into ulcers by secondary infection, irritant contact dermatitis, rubbing, and other trauma. The primary pustule of candidiasis or herpes simplex virus (HSV) infection, the primary vesicle in an acute eczematous process (contact dermatitis), or the primary bulla in bullous diseases or drug eruptions will all eventually rupture, resulting in erosions and/or ulcerative disease. Furthermore, an ulcerative lesion that is partially treated or healing may appear to be an erosion. Erosions usually heal without scarring, whereas ulcers, especially if large, deep, or long-standing, will likely result in scarring.

Patient history and physical examination provide important clues to the cause of a vulvar ulcer. Laboratory testing, however, is usually required for accurate diagnosis because the clinical presentation may be atypical due to compromised immunity, chronicity, severity, coexisting conditions, secondary infection, or secondary reactions to previous treatments. In 1 study, for example, diagnosis of a genital ulcer based on clinical examination correctly identified HSV in approximately 50% of cases, whereas the sensitivity of the clinical diagnosis for syphilis was 18%.[5]

Approach to the Patient, Evaluation, and Work-Up

As noted previously, vulvar ulcers are a nonspecific finding with many potential causes. Although the most common causes of vulvar ulcers in the United States are HSV and syphilis, the list of differential diagnoses in **Box 1** is purposefully comprehensive to emphasize the importance of a thorough assessment.

Initial screening laboratory tests for sexually active patients presenting with vulvar ulcers should focus on the common infectious causes and should include diagnostic testing for HSV (via viral culture or polymerase chain reaction [PCR]), serologic testing for syphilis (via rapid plasma reagin), bacterial culture, yeast culture, pregnancy testing, and screening for human immunodeficiency syndrome, as warranted. It is notable that HSV can be cultured from more than 90% of fluid-filled lesions, whereas ulcerations can be cultured only 70% of the time, and only 27% can be cultured at the crusted stage. PCR is 3 to 4 times more likely to isolate HSV than is viral culture.[6] Comprehensive care of sexually active patients with genital ulcers also includes screening for *Chlamydia trachomatis*, *Neisseria gonorrhoeae*, human immunodeficiency virus, and hepatitis B and C viruses, because many of these infections are asymptomatic.

Girls and women without history of sexual activity are typically screened in the same manner as sexually active patients due to concern of possible nondisclosure, misunderstanding of risk factors, and sexual abuse.

In cases of chronic or recurrent ulcers with negative screening for HSV and syphilis, additional evaluation and alternative diagnoses should be considered,[7] such as serology for Epstein-Barr virus, cytomegalovirus, and *Mycoplasma pneumoniae*. When the genital ulcers are unilateral and in a dermatomal distribution, testing for varicella-zoster virus should included as well.

The other sexually transmitted infections that cause genital ulcers, chancroid, granuloma inguinale, and lymphogranuloma venereum, are all quite uncommon in North America and can often be eliminated by a careful travel and sexual experience history.

The interview will usually elicit historical clues that can focus the differential diagnosis on trauma, drug reactions, contact dermatitis, and graft-versus-host disease as the cause. A biopsy is warranted when a dermatosis is suspected, for recurrent lesions without firm diagnosis, for any atypical findings, or for lesions suspicious for malignancy.

The best histologic findings will be found by biopsying the edge of the lesion, rather than the necrotic center. A wedge excision of the edge often gives the optimal specimen for the pathologist but may not be feasible. Alternatively, 2 smaller punch biopsies may suffice. It is critical to send the specimens, as well as a summary of the history and clinical findings and photograph as able, to a pathologist skilled in both gynecologic pathology and dermatopathology. If a bullous dermatosis is suspected, refer the patient to dermatology for biopsy, including standard hematoxylin-eosin stain and direct immunofluorescence.

While laboratory results are pending, symptomatic and supportive treatment should be directed toward pain relief, prevention of scarring, and specific treatment based on presumptive diagnosis:

1. Remove all irritants: soaps, OTC products, wet wipes, and so forth.
2. Counsel gentle vulvar skin care: using spray bottles with saline or voiding in the bath to reduce dysuria.
3. Restore the skin barrier: petrolatum or zinc oxide barrier after soak.
4. Administer pain control: lidocaine jelly 2% or lidocaine 5% ointment, nonsteroidal anti-inflammatory drugs, or narcotics, as warranted.
5. Consider acyclovir if primary HSV is the likely diagnosis.
6. Consider topical corticosteroid ointment if aphthous ulcers is the likely diagnosis.
7. Consider oral antibiotics if bacterial infection is suspected.
8. Consider consultation to dermatology as warranted.

All patients who may have a sexually transmitted infection should be advised to refrain from sexual activity while awaiting test results. Counseling regarding partner or contact testing and condom use is key to decreasing potential transmission. Follow-up should be arranged within 1 week of the initial visit to assess the clinical response to therapy and review results of diagnostic testing.

In summary, a focused, strategic approach to the clinical presentation of vulvar ulcers is recommended. If diagnosis remains elusive after a detailed history, examination, and laboratory studies, consider collaborating with a dermatologist for additional work up.

ACKNOWLEDGMENTS

The author gratefully acknowledges the substantial contribution of Kristin D. Thompson in preparing and editing this article.

REFERENCES

1. Edwards L, Lynch PJ, editors. Genital dermatology atlas. 2nd edition. Philadelphia: Lippincott Williams & Wilkins; 2011.
2. Black MM, Ambros-Rudolph C, Edwards L, et al. Obstetric and gynecologic dermatology. 3rd edition. Elsevier Limited; 2008.
3. Sehgal V, Pandhi D, Khurana A. Nonspecific genital ulcers. Clin Dermatol 2014; 32:259.
4. Gomes CM, Giraldo PC, Gomes Fde A, et al. Genital ulcers in women: clinical, microbiologic and histopathologic characteristics. Braz J Infect Dis 2007;11(2): 254–60.

5. Bogaerts J, Vuylsteke B, Martinez Tello W, et al. Simple algorithms for the management of genital ulcers: evaluation in a primary health care centre in Kigali, Rwanda. Bull World Health Organ 1995;73(6):761–7.
6. Wald A, Huang ML, Carrell D, et al. Polymerase chain reaction for detection of herpes simplex virus (HSV) DNA on mucosal surfaces: comparison with HSV isolation in cell culture. J Infect Dis 2003;188(9):1345–51.
7. Bandow GD. Diagnosis and management of vulvar ulcers. Dermatol Clin 2010; 28(4):753–64.

Challenging Ulcerative Vulvar Conditions

Hidradenitis Suppurativa, Crohn Disease, and Aphthous Ulcers

Kristen M.A. Stewart, MD

KEYWORDS

- Vulvar • Ulcer • Hidradenitis suppurativa • Crohn disease • Aphthous ulcers

KEY POINTS

- Hidradenitis suppurativa is a common condition that can be disabling and warrants early recognition and multimodal treatment.
- The vulvar lesions of metastatic Crohn disease present with a range of clinical findings and can precede the diagnosis of gastrointestinal symptoms by months to years.
- Aphthous ulcers are a clinical diagnosis of exclusion and can be classified as primary or secondary to systemic disease.

HIDRADENITIS SUPPURATIVA

Hidradenitis suppurativa (HS), also known as acne inversa, and historically as Verneuil's disease, is a common, chronic, disabling disease that unfortunately is often misdiagnosed and undertreated.[1] HS is an inflammatory cutaneous disease localized to intertriginous areas, including axillary, inguinal, anogenital, and inframammary skin. It is characterized by acute, recurrent, painful cysts and draining nodules, as well as chronic secondary scarring, dyspigmentation, and fistula formation.[2] The disease presents after puberty, commonly during young adulthood, and has a duration of many years, with periodic improvement and worsening of symptoms. HS has an estimated prevalence of 1% to 4%,[3,4] with a notable female-to-male predominance of 3:1.[5] The clinical spectrum can vary in severity from relatively mild cases with occasional inflammatory papulonodules to severe cases with frequent inflammatory lesions, ulcerative draining sinuses, and severe scarring. Regardless of severity, this disease has a significant impact on a patient's quality of life, personal relationships, and self-esteem.[6–8]

There are no financial disclosures or conflicts of interest to report.
Total Dermatology Care Center P.A., 915 West Monroe Street, Suite 101, Jacksonville, FL 32204, USA
E-mail address: kstewart@totaldermcare.com

Obstet Gynecol Clin N Am 44 (2017) 453–473
http://dx.doi.org/10.1016/j.ogc.2017.05.009
obgyn.theclinics.com

The pathogenesis of HS has not been completely elucidated yet and is likely multifactorial, involving a complex interplay among multiple contributing factors: a primary dysfunction of the folliculopilosebaceous unit, the individual's genetics and hormones, and immune dysregulation. The current fundamental theory is that HS is a disease of the folliculopilosebaceous unit attributed to defects in the follicular wall. Influenced by an individual's genetics and hormones, keratinocytes in the follicular epithelium hyperproliferate and sebum is increased, causing occlusion of the follicle. The follicle expands, eventually ruptures, and releases sebum, skin cells, and bacteria, triggering an intense inflammatory response. In HS patients, this acute reaction does not heal normally, but ultimately transforms into a chronic wound. Current theory holds that, as the body attempts to heal the inflammatory response, it instead entraps the sebum, skin cells, and bacteria from the ruptured follicle as well as stem cells found in the pilar unit, creating a buried invasive proliferative gelatinous mass (IPGM) and thereby producing the cysts, sinus tracts, and draining nodules characteristic of the disease.[9–13]

Several factors seem to contribute to the pathogenesis of HS, including genetic predisposition, smoking, diet, obesity, hormones, bacteria, immune factors, and inflammation. The influence of genetic susceptibility in HS is significant, with about 40% of patients having an affected family member.[14,15] Smoking is considered to be a contributing factor to HS, because, unlike controls, the majority of HS patients are smokers or have a history of smoking,[3] and studies have shown that HS symptoms improve when smoking is discontinued.[16] This correlation is not surprising, because nicotine is a known trigger of inflammation and may contribute to follicular plugging.

The potential contributions of diet, obesity, and hormones seem to be interwoven. Theories are adapted from acne studies, which have proposed that high glycemic load diets and dairy consumption may trigger relative androgen excess by increasing the sensitivity of androgen receptors on the folliculopilosebaceous unit, thereby promoting sebum production and follicular plugging.[17] These same dietary triggers also contribute to obesity, which has been theorized to increase shear stress on intertriginous skin, further promoting follicular occlusion.[3,18,19] The apparent relationship between androgens and HS is demonstrated by disease onset at menarche, and by observations that symptoms flare for many women premenstrually or with exposure to androgenic progestins and often improve during pregnancy and after menopause.[15,20] Further, antiandrogen treatment shows some benefit for both men and women. Additional studies are necessary to delineate the roles of diet, obesity, and hormones in HS.

Bacteria have been implicated in the pathogenesis, and antibiotics have been used as a treatment—although not a cure—with some success. That HS is not cured with antibiotics supports the current understanding that the role of bacteria is secondary. Most early, nonfluctuant lesions tend to be sterile, whereas fluctuant and chronic lesions are often polymicrobial and culture a wide variety of bacteria, including staphylococci, streptococci, Gram-negative rods, and anaerobic bacteria.[21–23] Acutely, bacterial contaminants from normal skin likely contribute to HS by stimulating the inflammatory response. Scarring and entrapment of a bacterial biofilm may explain the chronic inflammation associated with HS and its lack of response to antibiotic treatment.[24] Positive cultures are seen more frequently in suppurative, fluctuant nodules and may represent overgrowth of normal flora secondary to infection.

Recent HS research has focused on the role of immune factors and systemic inflammation.[25,26] The cutaneous inflammation of HS only very rarely produces systemic symptoms, such as fever and lymphadenopathy. HS has, however, been associated with the metabolic syndrome, which is defined by hypertension, diabetes, dyslipidemia, and abdominal obesity.[25–27] The prevalence of the metabolic syndrome in patients with HS has been estimated to be as high as 50%.[27] HS has also been linked to several autoimmune and systemic inflammatory conditions, such as inflammatory bowel disease and various arthropathies; to hormone-related disorders, such as polycystic ovarian syndrome and thyroid disease; to malignancies, such as squamous cell carcinoma; to pyoderma gangrenosum; and to psychological comorbidities, such as depression.[26–29]

History and Physical Examination

The diagnosis of HS is often delayed, likely due to a patient's hesitation to present for care, the episodic natural course of the disease, and frequent lack of continuity of care. Patients often present to urgent care centers and emergency departments with the complaint of "boils" or cysts, ingrown hairs, "staph" infections, and folliculitis. In these settings of fragmented care, a patient's history of recurrence and chronicity are easily missed, leading to a misdiagnosis of isolated abscess or folliculitis.[1] Alternatively, patients may present to primary care and gynecologists for routine care between flares when examination findings are less obvious, but the scarring stigmata of previous disease activity may still be evident. When such a patient presents, ask her one of these questions:

- Do you repeatedly have outbreaks of big, sore, or painful nodules or boils that heal with scars in any of these locations: armpits, groin, anal region, under the breasts, or in folds on the stomach or around the navel?
- Over the last 12 months, have you repeatedly had big, painful nodules or boils located in the armpits or in the groin, a disease called hidradenitis?[30]

Collect additional medical history including asking about family members with similar symptoms, tobacco abuse, symptoms associated with hyperandrogenism, polycystic ovarian syndrome, and insulin resistance.

The physical examination should include a whole-body mucocutaneous examination, focusing on the skin, oropharynx, anogenital areas, lymph nodes, and joints. Inspect the axilla, chest, inguinal creases, vulva, perineum, perianal skin, buttocks, and medial thighs for comedones, acneiform papules and pustules, inflammatory nodules, sinus tracts, ulcers, erosions, drainage, granulation tissue, induration, edema, lymphedema, lichenification, dyspigmentation, scars (atrophic, hypertrophic, keloidal), strictures, and contractures. Document the number, type, size, and distribution of such lesions as well as the presence or absence of lymphadenopathy and any associated findings, such as acne and pilonidal cysts.

Approach to the Patient: Evaluation and Workup

The diagnosis of HS is made using the following clinical criteria:

1. The presence of typical lesions (double, multiheaded, or tombstone comedones; deep-seated, painful, inflamed nodules; abscesses; sinus tracts with or without ulceration; and scarring);
2. Located in a characteristic distribution (axillae, inframammary chest, inguinal, and anogenital); and
3. Chronically relapsing and often recurrent in the same site(s).

Double, multiheaded, or tombstone comedones ("black heads") are characteristic of HS. Extensive inflammation and multiple recurrent nodules within a limited area may predispose the patient to the formation of linear and intercommunicating sinus tracts. Sinus tracts often express seropurulent, malodorous, bloody discharge and may ulcerate. Inflammatory lesions distributed on the lower abdominal wall, vulva, or perianal area can cause acute or chronic vulvar edema.

Healing or healed lesions can range in appearance from pink or skin-colored to hyperpigmented. Depending on the severity and duration of disease, the scars may range from discrete depressed, atrophic papulonodules or scars, to dense ropelike bands, to indurated plaques affecting the whole axillary or groin area. Severe scar bands and keloidal scars can cause contractures and impede mobility.

The inflammatory lesions of HS can usually be differentiated by clinical appearance and, if needed, bacterial culture. Unlike a furuncle, which is an infection of the hair follicle that can lead to an abscess, primary HS lesions are deep-seated and round-topped, and lack the pointed appearance of furuncles. Also unlike furuncles, cultures from HS lesions are usually negative or grow only nonpathogenic organisms; however, there are cases where an HS lesion becomes secondarily infected. Abscesses, furuncles, carbuncles, and folliculitis are transient lesions that should respond to appropriate antibiotic treatment and should not be associated with localized recurrence, the presence of multiple comedones, or the development of sinus tracts.

HS lesions must also be differentiated from metastatic Crohn disease (CD), anal fistulas, cellulitis, ischiorectal or perirectal abscesses, squamous cell carcinoma, deep fungal and mycobacterial infections, granuloma inguinale, lymphogranuloma venereum, noduloulcerative syphilis, Bartholin duct abscesses or cysts, and pilonidal cysts. Bacterial and tissue cultures are warranted in cases where a primary infection is suspected. Biopsy is warranted if CD is suspected, for atypical presentations, for recalcitrant disease, and for any lesions clinically suspicious for malignancy (the most common of which is squamous cell carcinoma).

Skin biopsies, cultures, laboratory tests, and radiologic imaging are usually not necessary for the diagnosis of HS. However, ultrasound imaging may be useful for staging and preoperative assessment of the subclinical extent of disease.

There are multiple systems used for staging HS (**Box 1**). The system used most frequently clinically – and historically used to guide treatment – is the Hurley staging system, which defines 3 stages of severity (**Figs. 1–3**).[31] The other staging systems can be used to assess treatment effectiveness. As none of theses staging systems directly accounts for quality-of-life measures that matter most to patients – pain, drainage, odor, and effect on jobs and personal relationships, this author recommends that these critical measures be quantified via the Dermatology Quality of Life Index.

Management

With the exception of recent randomized controlled studies of adalimumab, the majority of data in the literature regarding the treatment of HS are based on small case series and clinical experience. There are no uniform or standardized treatment plans. The current approach advocates early diagnosis and a comprehensive management plan that includes both supportive care and combined medical and surgical treatment tailored to the individual and escalated as warranted.

Active HS has a duration of many years, with periodic improvement and worsening of symptoms and long-term chronic sequelae.[15] Flares can be triggered by weight gain, stress, hormonal changes, heat, and perspiration. All treatment of HS should start with general measures, including education, referral to supportive resources, and control of potentially exacerbating factors. Patients should be educated and reassured that HS is neither contagious nor owing to poor hygiene and that the symptoms can be treated.[7] It is important to recognize the psychosocial impact on the patient and to offer quality resources, such as the Hidradenitis Suppurativa Foundation

---

Box 1
Staging systems of hidradenitis suppurativa[18,31,32]

1. The Hurley staging system describes 3 distinct clinical stages.
   - Stage I – solitary or multiple, isolated abscess formation without scarring or sinus tracts.
   - Stage II – recurrent abscesses, single or multiple widely separated lesions, with sinus tract formation.
   - Stage III – diffuse or broad involvement, with multiple interconnected sinus tracts and abscesses.

2. The Sartorius Hidradenitis Suppurativa Score is made by counting involved regions, nodules, and sinus tracts.
   - Anatomic region involved (axilla, groin, genital, gluteal, or other inflammatory region left and/or right): 3 points per region involved.
   - Number and scores of lesions (abscesses, nodules, fistulas, scars): 2 points for each nodule, 4 points for each fistula, 1 point for each scar, 1 point each for "other."
   - Longest distance between 2 relevant lesions (ie, nodules and fistulas in each region, or size if only 1 lesion): Less than 5 cm, 2 points; less than 10 cm, 4 points; more than 10 cm, 8 points.
   - Lesions clearly separated by normal skin in each region: If yes, 0 points; if no, 6 points.

3. The 6-point Physician Global Assessment ranges from clear to very severe. It is used in clinical trials to measure clinical improvement in inflammatory nodules, abscesses, and draining fistulae.

4. The Hidradenitis Suppurativa Clinical Response is defined as a 50%-or-greater reduction in inflammatory lesion count (abscesses and inflammatory nodules), and no increase in abscesses or draining fistulas when compared with baseline. This system has recently been used to assess the effectiveness of treatment with biologics.

5. It is also useful to consider the degree of pain, the number of flares, and the impact on daily life in hidradenitis suppurativa. The Cardiff Dermatology Life Quality Index questionnaire is often used.

(hsfoundation.org) and Hidradenitis Suppurativa USA (hs-usa.webs.com). As warranted, emphasize the importance of smoking cessation, diet, and weight loss on treatment outcomes by providing education and facilitating appropriate referrals.

Specifically address skin care by teaching the patient to maintain the skin barrier and to avoid skin trauma by not scrubbing, picking, or squeezing affected skin,

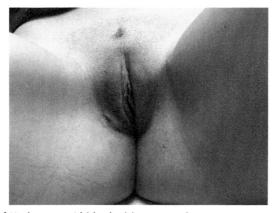

Fig. 1. Example of Hurley stage I hidradenitis suppurativa.

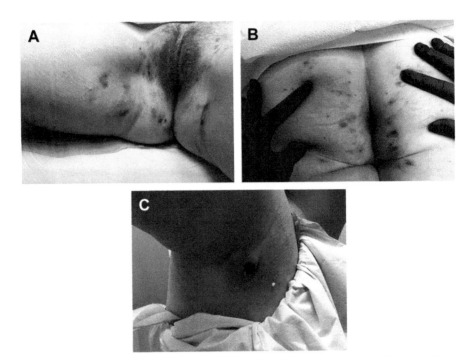

Fig. 2. Example of Hurley stage II hidradenitis suppurativa with multiple discrete and connected lesions with sinus tracts affecting (*A*) the vulva, inguinal creases, medial thighs, (*B*) buttocks and (*C*) axilla. Axillary ulcer with suppuration and granulation tissue.

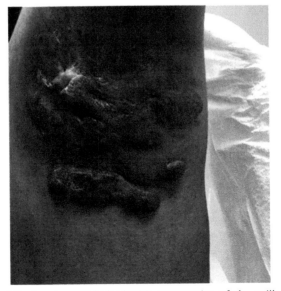

Fig. 3. Example of Hurley stage III hidradenitis suppurativa of the axilla, complicated by keloidal scarring.

wearing loose clothing, and avoiding excessive heat. If sweat is an irritant, consistently applying an over-the-counter clinical strength antiperspirant product nightly to the axilla and groin may help. The skin should be cleaned with a gentle cleanser. The patient should avoid consistent use of antiseptic cleansers that could lead to bacterial resistance, such as chlorhexidine gluconate. Benzoyl peroxide wash and zinc pyrithione-containing shampoos as well as dilute bleach baths (or hypochlorous acid spray or gel) may be considered to control odor and reduce bacterial colonization.[33,34]

Dressing HS lesions is inherently difficult due to the location in hair-bearing flexures, associated limb movement, friction from clothing, and sweat. For actively draining lesions, first apply petrolatum to prevent the bandage from sticking to the wound and then choose a nonadhesive dressing, as absorptive as necessary for the specific lesion, which can be fashioned to stay in place with undergarments or elastic fishnet.[33]

Like many other chronic, waxing and waning inflammatory conditions, HS requires a treatment plan that addresses:

1. Acute, short-term management of painful flares;
2. Long-term maintenance to reduce the incidence of inflamed nodules and prevent progression of disease and flares; and
3. Complications and sequelae, such as scarring, dyspigmentation, and sinus tract and fistula formation, as well as comorbidities.

Long-term maintenance treatment options usually require weeks to be effective, and therefore a distinct management plan for acute, painful flares is required. Surgical procedures, such as simple incision and drainage, which are appropriate for the treatment of traditional abscesses, should be avoided because HS lesions almost invariably recur, and such treatment may increase scarring.[35] Rather, in the case of focal, painful, fluctuant nodules, the affected area should be debrided using a deroofing technique as described below. This will not only allow for drainage and relief of acute pain, but also optimize healing and prevention of recurrence. Nonfluctuant HS nodules can be treated with intralesional injection of triamcinolone (0.1–0.5 mL of 5–10 mg/mL), which has been shown to decrease redness, size, edema, suppuration, and pain.[36] Additionally, short courses of a wide variety of antibiotics, such as a 7- to 14-day course of doxycycline or minocycline (100 mg twice daily) and amoxicillin with clavulanic acid (500 mg 3 times daily), have been used in an attempt to hasten the resolution of a flare. Additionally, short 1- to 2-week courses of prednisone may be used during severe flares of HS.

Choosing the appropriate long-term treatment strategy for HS patients can be difficult, because there is no consistently effective treatment or cure. The Hurley staging system can be used to guide the initial treatment, but it is important to tailor any HS treatment plan to the patient's individual needs and disease factors and to combine topical, systemic, and surgical modalities. A key concept of HS treatment is that additive or adjunctive combination treatment is standard. Additionally, it is imperative to treat early and to continuously reassess symptom control and sequelae as quantified by the patient's view of the impact of the disease and its treatment on her life.

Topical management may effectively control symptoms in mild HS and can also be used as adjuvant treatment in moderate to severe disease. Topical clindamycin phosphate 1% is considered a first-line treatment owing to few associated adverse effects, efficacy, low cost, and ease of use. One study, a small randomized controlled trial, found that topical administration of clindamycin reduced abscess, nodule, and pustule formation.[37] As has been long established in acne treatment guidelines, adding a topical benzoyl peroxide product to any topical or oral antibiotic treatment may be prudent to minimize the risk of developing antibiotic resistance.[38]

When HS symptoms are recalcitrant to topical treatments, oral antibiotics are prescribed commonly. Although use of antibiotics has demonstrated clinical improvement of symptoms, as noted, they do not cure HS. Symptomatic improvement is likely owing primarily to the antiinflammatory properties of the antibiotics. Typically, doxycycline or minocycline (50–100 mg twice daily) is prescribed for 2 to 4 months. A combination of oral rifampin and clindamycin (300 mg each, twice daily for up to 10 weeks) has been shown to substantively improve moderate and severe Physician Global Assessment or Hurley stage II HS lesions in several case series.[39,40] Multiple additional combinations of 2 to 3 oral and intravenous antibiotics have been described in the literature.[41] Notably, there is increasing concern regarding the risk of inducing antibiotic resistance, making long-term and repeated antibiotic treatment controversial.[42]

Treatment with the biologic tumor necrosis factor-alpha inhibitors adalimumab and infliximab have been used to treat HS.[43,44] Tumor necrosis factor-alpha inhibitors likely improve symptoms of HS by decreasing inflammation. Adalimumab is the only agent approved by the US Food and Drug Administration, and studies have shown that adalimumab can decrease abscess and inflammatory nodule counts and improve pain scores significantly.[44] Ideally, biologics should be started early in cases of moderate HS with the goal of minimizing scarring and the need for surgical intervention. Biologics may be used in combination with hormonal and antibiotic treatments and can be used as a pretreatment before surgical procedures.

The role of hormones on the pathogenesis and treatment of HS is not clear. Consider antiandrogen therapies in all women, especially those who also have diabetes, polycystic ovarian syndromes, or whose symptoms flare with menses. Oral contraceptive pills containing ethinyl estradiol and drospirenone, often in combination with spironolactone (50–125 mg daily), a synthetic steroid with antiandrogenic activity, are frequently used with success in woman with HS and have been shown to be more effective than antibiotics.[45] Metformin, a biguanide hypoglycemic medication, increases insulin sensitivity, which ultimately decreases the sensitivity of the androgen receptors.[46] Long-term use in HS patients, especially those who are obese or diabetic, has been advocated as medical management for metabolic control.[47]

Finasteride, a 5α-reductase inhibitor that is indicated to treat prostate cancer, has been reported in a few case reports to improve lesions in both men and women with HS.[48] Dutasteride has been reported anecdotally to improve HS in male patients.[47,49] These medications should be reserved for severe, recalcitrant cases and used judiciously in women, given their potential for teratogenicity.

Oral retinoid treatment may benefit HS patients by reducing ductal occlusion. Isotretinoin, although commonly successful in the treatment of recalcitrant acne, shows only limited efficacy in the treatment of HS.[50,51] However, a recent systematic review of etretinate (which is not available in the United States) and its metabolite acitretin found that 66% of treated patients had significant improvement of their HS lesions.[52] Pregnancy should be avoided for 1 month after isotretinoin treatment, and for 3 years after acitretin. Thus, the use of acitretin is typically avoided in women of childbearing potential.

Surgical intervention is a critical component of treating both the acute, individual flares of HS and the chronic sequelae and complications. As previously noted, the antibiotic-resistant IPGM that may persist in epithelialized nodules, fistulous tracts, and fibrotic scars can trigger the development of chronic wounds. The goal of surgical management, via variations of debridement and excision, is to remove any foreign material, IPGM, and scar tissue so that the wound can progress beyond the inflammatory stage toward healing, thereby limiting disease progression and preventing recurrence.[53,54]

Deroofing an HS lesion is a specific type of debridement, which can be accomplished by multiple methods, depending on the location and extent of disease. In the majority of cases, it can be performed in the office setting, sometimes over several visits, with local anesthesia. Medical management should be continued in combination with surgical treatment. In cases of severe disease, treatment with antibiotics, biologics, or prednisone to minimize inflammation before surgical treatment is recommended. Wide excision of the entire affected area or en bloc excision, with or without skin grafting and reconstruction, may be required for patients with chronic and extensive Hurley stage III disease and is beyond the scope of this article.

The core steps of deroofing HS lesions are as follows.

1. Remove the roof of each abscess, nodule, and sinus tract being treated.
2. Probe and explore the base and margins and expose any connections to other sinuses and nodules.
3. Completely remove all foreign material, including keratinaceous debris, seropurulent material, IPGM, and scar tissue.
4. Allow both small and large final defects to heal by secondary intent.[53,54]

Focal lesions smaller than 8 mm can be deroofed using cutaneous punch tool. Larger lesions can be deroofed using scissors, electrosurgery, or a CO_2 laser. Scissor tips or a malleable metal probe are used to probe and explore for connections. Remove all debris either by firmly scrubbing the base of the wound with coarse gauze or by using a curette (**Fig. 4**). Unrecognized connections and persistent foreign

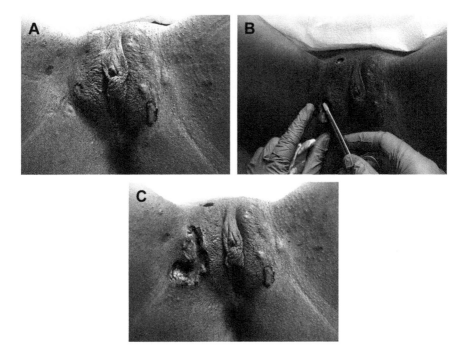

Fig. 4. Surgical debridement in a patient with Hurley stage II hidradenitis suppurativa. (*A*) Baseline, before debridement. (*B*) Punch excision of focal HS lesion on right mons and identification of sinus tracts of the right labium majus. (*C*) Hurley stage II immediate status after deroofing via punch excision on right mons and via scissor excision on right lateral labium majus.

material will interfere with healing and can trigger recurrence. Hemostasis is achieved with ferric chloride or aluminum chloride, and electrocautery is rarely needed. Typically, no additional debridement of the wound is needed during the healing phase.[54,55]

In the literature, wounds are cleansed gently and dressed once to twice daily with mupirocin or petrolatum ointment and covered with gauze or a simple bandage. It has been this author's recent practice to dress the wounds with Celacyn Prescription Scar Management Gel (Oculus Innovative Sciences, Inc., Petaluma, CA), which combines Microcyn technology—to stabilize nontoxic hypochlorous acid in a pH-neutral hydrogel—with dimethicone.

In an open study of 88 deroofed lesions in 44 consecutive patients with Hurley stage I or II disease, 83% did not show a recurrence after a median follow-up of 34 months. Of the treated patients, 90% would recommend the deroofing technique to other patients with HS.[53]

Adjunctive treatments that may have some benefit in treating HS include the following.

1. Hair laser removal: Therapy with the neodymium-doped yttrium aluminum garnet laser has been demonstrated to decrease HS lesion counts, possibly secondary to hair epilation and follicular deocclusion effects.[56,57]
2. Dietary supplements of zinc gluconate with cooper: Zinc is both an antiinflammatory and an antiandrogenic, inhibiting isoenzymes of 5α-reductase. Zinc gluconate (90 mg daily) yielded 8 complete and 14 partial remissions in 22 patients.[58]
3. Topical treatment with resorcinol: As a keratinolytic aimed at preventing follicular occlusion in HS patients, resorcinol has shown some benefit in 1 small study.[59]

The treatment of HS in pregnant women and women planning pregnancy is especially difficult, because all potentially teratogenic treatments must be discontinued, including hormonal treatments and many of the commonly used antibiotics.[20,60] In addition, although biologic therapies (infliximab, adalimumab) are pregnancy category B medications, their manufacturers advise discontinuation of treatment before a planned pregnancy. Consequently, medical treatment options for pregnant woman with HS are limited. Therefore, the use of topical treatments, intralesional corticosteroids, and surgical treatments such as deroofing, local or wide excision, and cryotherapy should be maximized as able.[20,60,61]

Regardless of where these patients initially present for their skin disease, a multidisciplinary approach that includes dermatology, gynecology, primary care, general and plastic surgery, and even subspecialties such as wound care, rheumatology, endocrinology, and psychiatry/psychology, should be used in the treatment of this heterogenous, multifactorial disease.

METASTATIC CROHN DISEASE OF THE VULVA

CD has classically been viewed as a chronic inflammatory bowel disease that is characterized by segmental noncaseating granulomas and may affect any portion of the gastrointestinal (GI) tract, from the mouth to the anus. The current paradigm has broadened the view of this disease to a multisystem inflammatory disorder with the potential to affect multiple organs, including the skin.[62]

CD usually begins during the second or third decade of life and has a slight female predominance. GI CD commonly presents with symptoms of abdominal pain, diarrhea, malabsorption, and weight loss. There can be fever, rectal bleeding, anal fissures, and perirectal abscesses. Along with the characteristic GI findings of this disease, patients with CD may also present with manifestations outside the GI tract, including ocular findings, arthritis, and mucocutaneous lesions.[63,64]

Mucosal and skin lesions are the most common manifestations of CD outside the GI tract, occurring in up to 44% of patients.[64] The mucosal and skin findings of CD can be classified as CD-specific lesions, which histologically demonstrate granulomatous inflammation indistinguishable from GI lesions; reactive lesions associated with CD, such as erythema nodosum and oral aphthae; and associated lesions, which develop as a consequence of the disease or its management, such as nutritional deficiency and adverse effects of treatment.[62–64]

CD-specific granulomatous lesions that extend directly from the GI tract, such as perianal skin tags, perianal and peristomal fistulas, perineal ulceration, and oral disease, are the most common of the mucocutaneous manifestations of CD.[64] Parks and colleagues[65] were the first to describe cutaneous granulomatous lesions, histologically identical to those found in the intestines, occurring at sites separate from the GI tract. Although this entity is known as metastatic CD (MCD), Laftah and colleagues[66] suggest that such lesions might better be described as "noncontiguous" lesions, because there is no link to malignancy.

MCD can occur on any skin surface, but has a predilection for inguinal, perineal, and vulvar skin folds, and should be considered in the differential diagnosis of vulvar ulcers and vulvar edema.[67] Owing to its infrequent incidence, nonspecific clinical findings, and variable timing in relation to GI CD, MCD can be difficult to diagnose.[68] This section reviews the clinical features, histopathologic findings, differential diagnosis, and treatment options for vulvar MCD.

History and Physical Examination

Patients with vulvar MCD may present to various physicians, including internists, gynecologists, gastroenterologists, and dermatologists, with any variety of complaints, such as vaginal discharge, painful ulcerations, genital pruritus, and dyspareunia. MCD can be misdiagnosed initially as contact dermatitis, HS, and various sexually transmitted diseases. The medical interview should discern recent sexual exposure history, history of immunosuppression, GI symptoms, joint pain, and last menstrual period.

The vulvar lesions of MCD may present with a range of clinical findings, including labial edema, erythema, swelling, induration, or hypertrophy, which is often unilateral and can affect the labia majora and/or labia minora; vulvar ulcers, which can be focal or multiple, superficial, deep, or knife cut; exophytic, pseudocondylomatous, hypertrophic lesions, attributed to chronic inflammation and impaired lymphatic drainage; and fluctuant nodules or abscesses.[69–72] The physical examination should include an examination of the axillae and the breasts for stigmata of HS. MCD abscesses typically progress to ulcers with undermined edges, draining sinuses, and fistulae, resulting in scarring that can extend onto the mons, perineum, and inguinal creases and has the potential to be disfiguring and destructive.[69–72] Therefore, early diagnosis and timely management are important.

Approach to the Patient: Evaluation and Workup

The diagnosis of cutaneous CD is generally obvious if the patient has associated GI and perianal manifestations. MCD lesions most often occur at the same time or after a diagnosis of GI CD is made. Clinicians must be aware, however, that MCD can precede the diagnosis of GI CD by months to years. When MCD is diagnosed without GI involvement, subsequent onset of GI CD is most likely to occur within 2 months to 4 years in adults and 9 months to 14 years in children. In 1 review of 55 vulvar MCD cases, 25% of patients did not have any previous GI symptoms and had not been diagnosed with CD at the time of their vulvar symptoms.[70] Consequently, clinicians should keep vulvar MCD in the differential diagnosis of vulvar ulcers, vulvar edema, and vulvar nodules, even in the absence of a history of CD or abdominal complaints. Furthermore, vulvar CD can occur many years after a subtotal colectomy in patients with no evidence of other CD and can persist despite excision of intestinal disease or during a period of quiescent GI disease.[69]

Cutaneous CD should be suspected in patients with knife cut ulcers in the skin folds, aphthous ulcers, genital abscesses, scarring, perianal disease with swelling, fissures, anal and perineal tags, and in cases of rectovaginal fistulae developing after vaginal delivery. Fistulae associated with CD are often surrounded by granulation tissue along the edges, forming slightly friable, red nodules that may obscure tracts and imitate the appearance of HS. Consult with a gastroenterologist or colorectal surgeon and image as warranted to rule out possible enterocutaneous fistulae. The physical examination should include an examination of the axillae and the breasts for stigmata of HS.

As noted in the HS section of this article, the clinical differential diagnosis should be broad in all cases of nonspecific skin findings. Sexually transmitted infections should be ruled out. Knife cut linear erosions and ulcers, which resemble lacerations, are highly characteristic of MCD and are considered by some to be pathognomonic for the disease (**Fig. 5**). However, this clinical finding has also been reported in cutaneous tuberculosis and in linear erosive herpes simplex virus infection, which can be seen in immunocompromised patients.[72]

A biopsy of the affected skin showing granulomatous inflammation on histopathology strongly supports a diagnosis of MCD; however, histopathology is often nonspecific. In a 2011 case series, Foo and colleagues[71] observed that, because only approximately one-half of the patients diagnosed with GI CD demonstrate classic noncaseating granulomas in intestinal biopsies. Consequently, relying on this histopathologic finding to diagnose vulvar MCD definitively may result in misdiagnosis and underreporting. On the other hand, a pattern of granulomatous inflammation

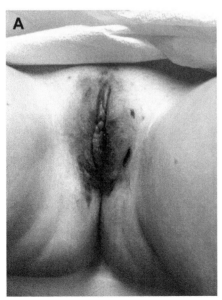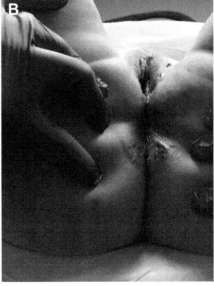

Fig. 5. Case of metastatic Crohn disease notable for (*A*) a knife cut ulcer, smaller punched out labial ulcers as well as (*B*) perianal ulcers.

also can be seen in sarcoidosis, mycobacterial infections, deep fungal infections, granuloma inguinale, foreign body reactions, and HS. Therefore, in patients without known GI CD, further workup to distinguished these conditions is warranted and should include ACE level, tissue culture, polarizing microscopy, and screening for tuberculosis with either an intradermal tuberculin reaction or QuaniFERON-TB Gold (Qiagen, Hilden, Germany) and chest radiographs. The clinical differential diagnosis also includes abscess of a Bartholin cyst, cellulitis, fistula, chronic lymphedema resulting from obstruction, Langerhans cell histiocytosis, erythema nodosum, pyoderma gangrenosum, intertrigo, and metastasis.

Management

Without treatment, lesions of MCD are chronic and can be a source of significant scarring, disfigurement, morbidity, and decreased quality of life. The severity of MCD does not always correlate with the severity of the underlying GI CD. Given the rarity of the condition and lack of prospective trials, there are no specific guidelines for the medical or surgical treatment of MCD. Kurtzman and colleagues[67] proposed an algorithmic approach to the management of MCD that is an excellent resource.

Mild, localized, or single MCD lesions may be treated successfully with potent to superpotent topical corticosteroids or steroid-sparing topical calcineurin inhibitors, such as tacrolimus ointment. These topical treatments, as well as intralesional triamcinolone acetonide (Kenalog) injections, can be used as monotherapy or combined with any other treatment. If symptoms are not well controlled, adding oral metronidazole (800–1500 mg daily, for at least 4 months) has been effective. In cases of more extensive or recalcitrant vulvar MCD, systemic glucocorticosteroids can be added.[67] To avoid long-term side effects, the dose should be tapered gradually to the least amount needed to control symptoms. Treatment with oral metronidazole alone or in combination with steroids has been shown to have a success rate of 87.5%.[70]

If systemic corticosteroids do not control symptoms or cannot be tapered, alternative systemic treatments should be considered. Systemic treatments for MCD include many of the same treatments used for GI CD. Specifically, tumor necrosis factor-alpha inhibitors have been shown to sustain remission of both GI CD and MCD.[73] Alternative immunosuppressants, such as azathioprine, methotrexate, cyclosporine, and thalidomide, have also been used successfully to treat MCD.[74] If monotherapy fails to control symptoms, various combinations of these agents may be used.

Vulvar MCD that is refractory to medical therapy or disfiguring may be treated surgically via vulvectomy, laser, or excision[67]; however, there is a significant risk of recurrence and poor wound healing. Long-term treatment and care of patients with vulvar MCD should include increased gynecologic surveillance due to the association between CD and vulvar intraepithelial neoplasia and address the psychological impact of the disease on quality of life.

VULVAR APHTHOUS ULCERS

Aphthae are painful, shallow ulcers that commonly occur on the oral mucosa and less commonly occur on the genital mucosa. The etiology of aphthae is unclear, but risk factors include stress, infections, hormonal factors, vitamin deficiency, and family history.[75] The diagnosis of complex aphthosis is challenging for the clinician, because it is a clinical diagnosis of exclusion, and is complicated generally by the broad differential diagnosis of genital ulcers. Moreover, it is frequently missed owing to assumption of sexually transmitted infection as the cause. Finally, as with all vulvar ulcers, it is universally distressing to the patient.

Aphthosis occurs in 2 forms: simple and complex. The recurrent small oral ulcers of simple aphthosis, commonly known as canker sores, affect 20% of the general population[76] and are generally recognized as troublesome, but benign. Complex aphthosis, in contrast, is rare and presents as either persistent, chronic oral aphthae or aphthae located on the oral and genital mucous membranes.[77]

Complex aphthosis can be classified as primary (ie, idiopathic with no identifiable underlying cause) or secondary to systemic disease. Secondary complex aphthosis arises in multiple circumstances: it may be associated with underlying systemic disease or syndromes; it may occur as a result of hematologic abnormalities; it can be triggered by medications; or it may be a reaction to an acute illness (**Box 2**).

A unique subset of reactive aphthosis occurs in non–sexually active girls and young woman who develop vulvar and oral ulcers in association with a fever and/or systemic illness.[82–85] Historically known as Lipschutz ulcer, ulcus vulvae acutum, and acute genital ulceration, Lehman and colleagues[82] later descriptively termed this specific cohort "reactive non–sexually related acute genital ulcers" to emphasize the likely etiology that the lesions result from an exuberant systemic immune response to acute infection. Multiple bacterial and viral infections have been associated with reactive non–sexually related acute genital ulcers.[84] Reactive non–sexually related acute genital ulcers are underrecognized by health care providers and should be considered in cases of acute vulvar ulcers in otherwise healthy adolescent girls without a sexual history and with a preceding fever or other acute systemic symptoms.

Box 2
Categories of aphthosis

I. Simple aphthosis

II. Complex aphthosis
  a. Primary, idiopathic complex aphthosis
  b. Secondary complex aphthosis
    i. Associated with underlying systemic disease
      1. Behçets disease
      2. Celiac disease
      3. Inflammatory bowel disease (Crohn disease and ulcerative colitis),
      4. Immunodeficiencies (including human immunodeficiency virus)
    ii. Associated with syndromes
      1. Sweet's syndrome
      2. Mouth and genital ulcers inflamed cartilage syndrome
      3. Periodic fever, aphthosis or pharyngitis, and adenitis syndrome
    iii. Hematologic abnormalities
      1. Hematinic deficiencies (iron, zinc, folate, and vitamins B_1, B_2, B_6, B_{12})
      2. Cyclic neutropenia
      3. Myeloproliferative disease
      4. Lymphopenia
    iv. Medications
      1. Nonsteroidal antiinflammatory drugs
      2. Nicorandil (a potassium channel activator)
    v. Reactive – response to an acute illness or infection
      1. Epstein–Bar virus
      2. Cytomegalovirus
      3. Influenza
      4. Group A streptococci
      5. *Mycoplasma pneumoniae*
      6. Lyme disease

Data from Refs.[78–82]

History and Physical Examination

A careful history should elucidate a description, onset, and duration of symptoms, history of any previous episodes of oral or vulvar lesions, age of menarche, assessment of sexual experience, potential triggers such as trauma or abuse, and all home treatments and medical treatments before presentation. Review potential systemic symptoms such as dysuria, fever, headache, malaise, arthralgia, anorexia, nausea, diarrhea, skin rash, sore throat, rhinorrhea, and cough, as well as ocular and neurologic symptoms. Inquire about a personal and family history of Behçets disease (BD), celiac disease, and CD.

The physical examination should include a full skin examination focused on the ocular, oral, and genital mucosa. Aphthae typically are single or multiple, painful, ovoid ulcers, with a clean or fibrinous yellow-to-gray base and surrounding erythematous halo, but can be necrotic. There are 3 main ulcer morphologies: minor aphthous ulcers are usually less than 5 mm in diameter, heal within 1 to 2 weeks, and account for about 80% of aphthous ulcer cases; major aphthous ulcers are larger (greater than 10 mm), take weeks or months to heal, and often leave scarring; and herpetiform ulcers are multiple pinpoint ulcers that heal within a month (**Fig. 6**). In general, the ulcers seen in aphthosis and BD are typically larger and less painful than lesions caused by herpes simplex virus. Edema of the labia is commonly seen with aphthous ulcers and can be severe.

Approach to the Patient: Evaluation and Workup

The diagnosis of vulvar aphthae is based on the history, clinical findings, and exclusion of other causes. Therefore, the evaluation depends on the identification of secondary

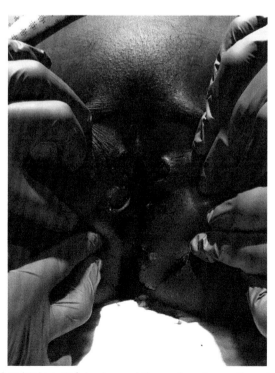

Fig. 6. Example of multiple, painful vulvar aphthous ulcers in an otherwise healthy preteen girl.

factors and, importantly, the exclusion of BD. Letsinger and colleagues[81] developed an evaluation algorithm that is an excellent resource.

Laboratory testing should be tailored to the individual patient and should routinely include polymerase chain reaction testing to rule out herpes simplex virus. Additional serologies for syphilis and human immunodeficiency virus should be added as appropriate. Biopsy results are nonspecific, but may be necessitated in some cases to rule out other pathology. Bacterial culture and either a potassium hydroxide preparation or fungal culture are only needed on a case-by-case basis to exclude secondary bacterial infection and occult local yeast. Although routine screening for potential infectious triggers of acute vulvar ulcers rarely alters management, the following screening may be warranted in some cases: serology for Epstein–Bar virus, cytomegalovirus, and *Mycoplasma pneumoniae*; polymerase chain reaction for influenza; and Antistreptolysin O and Lyme titers.

Recurrent oral and genital lesions characterize both BD and complex aphthosis. Unlike complex aphthosis, however, BD is a multisystem disease. As recognized by the International Study Group criteria published in 1990, there are no pathognomonic laboratory tests for BD.[82] In the absence of other systemic diseases, many experts diagnose BD in patients with recurrent oral aphthae (defined as occurring at least 3 times in 1 year) plus 2 of the following clinical features:

1. Recurrent genital aphthae (aphthous ulceration or scarring);
2. Eye lesions (including anterior or posterior uveitis, cells in vitreous on slit lamp examination, or retinal vasculitis observed by an ophthalmologist);
3. Skin lesions (including erythema nodosum, pseudovasculitis, papulopustular lesions, or acneiform nodules consistent with BD); and
4. A positive pathergy test (defined by a papule 2 mm or more in size developing 24 to 48 hours after oblique insertion of a 20-gauge needle 5 mm into the skin; generally performed on the forearm).

Although it is controversial, some have considered complex aphthosis a forme fruste of BD.[77] Although the vast majority of patients with complex aphthosis do not have and will not develop BD, complex aphthosis patients should be followed continuously to assess for evolution of BD owing to the potential morbidity associated with that disease.[77–80]

In cases of recurrent or chronic aphthae, rule out hematologic abnormalities caused by nutritional deficiencies and neutropenia with complete blood counts and testing of serum iron, folate, vitamin B_{12}, and zinc levels; consult with gastroenterology for evaluation of occult inflammatory bowel or celiac disease; and consult with ophthalmology, rheumatology, and neurology to rule out BD as warranted.[81]

Management

Patients and parents should be reassured that vulvar aphthae are analogous to oral canker sores and neither contagious nor sexually transmitted. Although there is no cure, the goals of treatments are to manage pain, speed healing, and reduce recurrence.

All patients should be educated on gentle skin and wound care that includes Sitz baths with plain warm water to clean and debride ulcers. Soaps, cleansers, and over-the-counter products should be avoided. Pain can be controlled with local anesthetics (eg, lidocaine 2% jelly or 5% ointment) and oral analgesics such as acetaminophen, nonsteroidal antiinflammatory drugs, and narcotics as needed. Occasionally, patients require hospitalization for placement of a urinary catheter and/or pain control.

The literature only contains low-level evidence regarding the treatment of complex aphthosis. Class 1 topical corticosteroids such as clobetasol propionate ointment are considered first-line treatment in complex aphthosis and can be combined with topical anesthetics.[81,86] Tacrolimus ointment is a topical calcineurin inhibitor and can replace clobetasol ointment as a steroid-sparing agent. Triamcinolone acetonide (5 mg/mL) can be injected into larger ulcers and ulcers that do not respond to topical steroids. Despite the theoretic risk of exacerbating a recent or current infection, short courses (5–14 days) of systemic corticosteroids can give symptomatic relief during acute, painful episodes. Systemic corticosteroids do not, however, affect the disease course, and ongoing treatment is not recommended due to the adverse side effects of long-term use.[81]

The traditional therapeutic ladder for complex aphthosis begins with systemic therapy with colchicine or dapsone.[80,86] A synergistic effect has been observed when these 2 drugs are used together. Lynde and colleagues[86] advocate additive therapies rather than replacing one monotherapy for another. Therefore, the second step in systemic treatment continues with these agents combined. It is notable that, in 2013, Dixit and colleagues[87] successfully used subantimicrobial dosing of doxycycline as an alternative steroid-sparing antiinflammatory agent in a small case series of patients with vulvar ulcers. Patients with recalcitrant disease are next treated with thalidomide.[80,87]

ACKNOWLEDGMENTS

The author gratefully acknowledges the substantial contribution of Kristin D. Thompson in preparing and editing this article.

REFERENCES

1. Saunte G, Boer J, Stratigos A. Diagnostic delay in hidradenitis suppurativa is a global problem. Br J Dermatol 2015;173(6):1546–9.
2. Revuz J. Hidradenitis suppurativa. J Eur Acad Dermatol Venereol 2009;23(9): 985–98.
3. Revuz JE, Canoui-Poitrine F, Wolkenstein P, et al. Prevalence and factors associated with hidradenitis suppurativa: results from two case-control studies. J Am Acad Dermatol 2008;59:596–601.
4. Jemec GB, Heidenheim M, Nielsen NH. The prevalence of hidradenitis suppurativa and its potential precursor lesions. J Am Acad Dermatol 1996;35(2, pt 1): 191–4.
5. Jemec GB. Hidradenitis suppurativa. N Engl J Med 2012;366:158–64.
6. Matusiak L, Bieniek A, Szepietwoski JC. Hidradenitis suppurativa markedly decreases quality of life and professional activity. J Am Acad Dermatol 2010;62: 706–8.
7. Esmann S, Jemec GB. Psychosocial impact of hidradenitis suppurativa: a qualitative study. Acta Derm Venereol 2011;91(3):328–32.
8. Kurek A, Peters EM, Chanwangpong A, et al. Profound disturbances of sexual health in patients with acne inversa. J Am Acad Dermatol 2012;67(3):422–8, 428.e1.
9. Nazary M, van der Zee HH, Prens EP, et al. Pathogenesis and pharmacotherapy of hidradenitis suppurativa. Eur J Pharmacol 2011;672:1.
10. von Laffert M, Helmbold P, Wohlrab J, et al. Hidradenitis suppurativa (acne inversa): early inflammatory events at terminal follicles and at interfollicular epidermis. Exp Dermatol 2010;19:533.

11. Danby FW, Jemec GB, Marsch WCh, et al. Preliminary findings suggest hidradenitis suppurativa may be due to defective follicular support. Br J Dermatol 2013; 168:1034.
12. Gniadecki R, Jemec GB. Lipid raft-enriched stem cell-like keratinocytes in the epidermis, hair follicles and sinus tracts in hidradenitis suppurativa. Exp Dermatol 2004;13:361.
13. Kurzen H, Kurokawa I, Jemec GB, et al. What causes hidradenitis suppurativa? Exp Dermatol 2008;17:455.
14. Fitzsimmons JS, Guilbert PR. A family study of hidradenitis suppurativa. J Med Genet 1985;22:367–73.
15. von der Werth JM, Williams HC. The natural history of hidradenitis suppurativa. J Eur Acad Dermatol Venereol 2000;14:389.
16. Denny G, Anadkat MJ. The effect of smoking and age on the response to first-line therapy of hidradenitis suppurativa: an institutional retrospective cohort study. J Am Acad Dermatol 2017;76(1):54–9.
17. Danby FW. Diet in the prevention of hidradenitis suppurativa (acne inversa). J Am Acad Dermatol 2015;73:S52.
18. Sartorius K, Emtestam L, Jemec GBE, et al. Objective scoring of hidradenitis suppurativa reflecting the role of tobacco smoking and obesity. Br J Dermatol 2009; 161(4):831–9.
19. Canoui-Poitrine F, Revuz JE, Wolkenstein P, et al. Clinical characteristics of a series of 302 French patients with hidradenitis suppurativa, with an analysis of factors associated with disease severity. J Am Acad Dermatol 2009;61:51–7.
20. Vossen AR, van Straalen KR, Prens EP, et al. Menses and pregnancy affect symptoms in hidradenitis suppurativa: a cross-sectional study. J Am Acad Dermatol 2017;76(Issue 1):155–6.
21. Sartorius K, Killasli H, Oprica C, et al. Bacteriology of hidradenitis suppurativa exacerbations and deep tissue cultures obtained during carbon dioxide laser treatment. Br J Dermatol 2012;166:879.
22. Nikolakis G, Join-Lambert O, Karagiannidis I, et al. Bacteriology of hidradenitis suppurativa/acne inversa: a review. J Am Acad Dermatol 2015;73(5 Suppl 1): S12–8.
23. Ring HC, Riis Mikkelsen P, Miller IM, et al. The bacteriology of hidradenitis suppurativa: a systematic review. Exp Dermatol 2015;24(10):727–31.
24. Kathju S, Lasko LA, Stoodley P. Considering hidradenitis suppurativa as a bacterial biofilm disease. FEMS Immunol Med Microbiol 2012;65:385.
25. Dessinioti C, Katsambas A, Antoniou C. Hidradenitis suppurativa (acne inversa) as a systemic disease. Clin Dermatol 2014;32(3):397–408.
26. Shlyankevich J, Chen AJ, Kim GE, et al. Hidradenitis suppurativa is a systemic disease with substantial comorbidity burden: a chart-verified case-control analysis. J Am Acad Dermatol 2014;71:1144–50.
27. Gold DA, Reeder VJ, Mahan MG, et al. The prevalence of metabolic syndrome in patients with hidradenitis suppurativa. J Am Acad Dermatol 2014;70(4):699–703.
28. Deckers IE, Benhadou F, Koldijk MJ. Inflammatory bowel disease is associated with hidradenitis suppurativa: results from a multicenter cross-sectional study. J Am Acad Dermatol 2017;76:49–53.
29. van der Zee HH, de Winter K, van der Woude CJ, et al. The prevalence of hidradenitis suppurativa in 1093 patients with inflammatory bowel disease. Br J Dermatol 2014;171(3):673–5.

30. Esmann S, Dufour DN, Jemec GB. Questionnaire-based diagnosis of hidradenitis suppurativa: specificity, sensitivity and positive predictive value of specific diagnostic questions. Br J Dermatol 2010;163:102–6.

31. Hurley H J. Axillary hyperhidrosis, apocrine bromhidrosis, hidradenitis suppurativa, and familial benign pemphigus: surgical approach. In: Roenigk RK, Roenigk HH, editors. Dermatologic surgery. New York: Dekker; 1989. p. 729.

32. Sartorius K, Lapins J, Emtestam L, et al. Suggestions for uniform outcome variables when reporting treatment effects in hidradenitis suppurativa. Br J Dermatol 2003;149:211–3.

33. Afsaneh A, Kirsner R. Local wound care and topical management of hidradenitis suppurativa. J Am Acad Dermatol 2015;73:S55–61.

34. Danesh MJ, Kimball A. Pyrithione zinc as a general management strategy for hidradenitis suppurativa. J Am Acad Dermatol 2015;73(5):e175.

35. Jemec GB. Clinical practice. Hidradenitis suppurativa. N Engl J Med 2012;366:158–64.

36. Riis P, Boer J, Prens E, et al. Intralesional triamcinolone for flares of hidradenitis suppurativa (HS): a case series. J Am Acad Dermatol 2016;75:1151–5.

37. Clemmensen OJ. Topical treatment of hidradenitis suppurativa with clindamycin. Int J Dermatol 1983;22(5):325–8.

38. Leyden JJ, Del Rosso JQ, Webster GF. Clinical considerations in the treatment of acne vulgaris and other inflammatory skin disorders: a status report. Dermatol Clin 2009;27:1.

39. Gener G, Canoui-Poitrine F, Revuz JE, et al. Combination therapy with clindamycin and rifampin for hidradenitis suppurativa: a series of 116 consecutive patients. Dermatology 2009;219:148–54.

40. van der Zee HH, Boer J, Prens EP, et al. The effect of combined treatment with oral clindamycin and oral rifampin in patience with hidradenitis suppurativa. Dermatology 2009;219:143–7.

41. Join-Lambert O, Coignard H, Jais JP, et al. Efficacy of rifampin-moxifloxacin-metronidazole combination therapy in hidradenitis suppurativa. Dermatology 2011;222:49–58.

42. Fischer AH, Haskin A, Okoye MD. Patterns of antimicrobial resistance in lesions of hidradenitis suppurativa. J Am Acad Dermatol 2017;76(2):309–13.e2.

43. Kimball AB, Okun MM, Williams DA, et al. Two phase 3 trials of adalimumab for hidradenitis suppurativa. N Engl J Med 2016;375:422–34.

44. Kimball AB, Kerdel F, Adams D, et al. Adalimumab for the treatment of moderate to severe hidradenitis suppurativa: a parallel randomized trial. Ann Intern Med 2012;157:846–55.

45. Kraft JN, Searles GE. Hidradenitis suppurativa in 64 female patients: retrospective study comparing oral antibiotics and antiandrogen therapy. J Cutan Med Surg 2007;11(4):125–31.

46. Verdolini R, Clayton N, Smith A, et al. Metformin for the treatment of hidradenitis suppurativa: a little help along the way. J Eur Acad Dermatol Venereol 2013;27(9):1101–8.

47. Margesson LJ, Danby FW. Hidradenitis suppurativa. Best Pract Res Clin Obstet Gynaecol 2014;28:1013–27.

48. Khandalavala BN, Do MV. Finasteride in hidradenitis suppurativa: a "male" therapy for a predominantly "female" disease. J Clin Aesthet Dermatol 2016;9(6):44–50.

49. Scheinfeld Noah. Hidradenitis suppurativa: a practical review of possible medical treatments based on over 350 hidradenitis patients. Dermatol Online J 2013; 19(4):1.

50. Gulliver W, Zouboulis CC, Prens E, et al. Evidence-based approach to the treatment of hidradenitis suppurativa/acne inversa, based on the European guidelines for hidradenitis suppurativa. Rev Endocr Metab Disord 2016;17(3):343–51.

51. Soria A, Canoui-Poitrine F, Wolkenstein P, et al. Absence of efficacy of oral isotretinoin in hidradenitis suppurativa: a retrospective study based on patients' outcome assessment. Dermatology 2009;218:134–5.

52. Boer J, Nazary M. Long-term results of acitretin therapy for hidradenitis suppurativa. Is acne inversa also a misnomer? Br J Dermatol 2011;164:170–5.

53. van der Zee HH, Prens EP, Boer J. Deroofing: a tissue-saving surgical technique for the treatment of mild to moderate hidradenitis suppurativa lesions. J Am Acad Dermatol 2010;63:475–80.

54. Danby F, Hazen P, Boer J. New and traditional surgical approaches to hidradenitis suppurativa. J Am Acad Dermatol 2015;73:S62–5.

55. Kohorst J, Baum C, Otley CC, et al. Surgical management of hidradenitis suppurativa: outcomes of 590 consecutive patients. Dermatol Surg 2016;42:1030–40.

56. Mahmoud BH, Tierney E, Hexsel C, et al. Prospective controlled clinical and histopathologic study of hidradenitis suppurativa treated with the long-pulsed neodymium:yttrium-aluminium-garnet laser. J Am Acad Dermatol 2010;62:637–45.

57. Tierney E, Mahmoud B, Hexsel C, et al. Randomized controlled trial for the treatment of HS with a neodymium-doped yttrium aluminium garnet laser. Dermatol Surg 2009;35:1188–98.

58. Brocard A, Knol A, Khammari A, et al. Hidradenitis suppurativa and zinc: a new therapeutic approach. a pilot study. Dermatology 2007;214:325.

59. Boer J, Jemec GB. Resorcinol peels as a possible self-treatment of painful nodules in hidradenitis suppurativa. Clin Exp Dermatol 2010;35:36.

60. Perng P, Zampella JG, Okoye GA. Management of hidradenitis suppurativa in pregnancy. J Am Acad Dermatol 2017;76(5):979–89.

61. Calogero P, Fabrizi G, Feliciani C, et al. Cryoinsufflation for Hurley Stage II Hidradenitis Suppurativa: a useful treatment option when systemic therapies should be avoided. JAMA Dermatol 2014;150(7):765–6.

62. Marzano AV, Borghi A, Stadnicki A, et al. Cutaneous manifestations in patients with inflammatory bowel diseases: pathophysiology, clinical features, and therapy. Inflamm Bowel Dis 2014;20(1):213–27.

63. Thrash M, Patel K, Shah C, et al. Cutaneous manifestations of gastrointestinal disease. J Am Acad Dermatol 2013;68:211.e1-33.

64. Lester LU, Rapinis RP. Dermatologic manifestations of colonic disorders. Curr Opin Gastroenterol 2008;25(1):66–73.

65. Parks A, Morson B, Pegum J. Crohn's disease with cutaneous involvement. Proc R Soc Med 1965;58:241–2.

66. Laftah Z, Bailey C, Zaheri S, et al. Vulval Crohn's disease: a clinical study of 22 patients. J Crohn's Colitis 2015;9(4):318–25.

67. Kurtzman D, Jones T, Lian F, et al. Metastatic Crohn's disease: a review and approach to therapy. J Am Acad Dermatol 2014;71:804–13.

68. Urbanek M, Neill SM, McKee PH. Vulval Crohn's disease: difficulties in diagnosis. Clin Exp Dermatol 1996;21:211–4.

69. Barrett M, de Parades V, Battistella M, et al. Crohn's disease of the vulva. J Crohn's Colitis 2014;8:563–70.

70. Andreani SM, Ratnasingham K, Dang HH, et al. Crohn's disease of the vulva. Int J Surg 2010;8(1):2–5.
71. Foo WC, Papalas JA, Robboy SJ, et al. Vulvar manifestations of Crohn's disease. Am J Dermatopathol 2011;33(6):588–93.
72. Ezzine-Sebai N, Fazaa B, Zeglaoui F, et al. Chronic linear ulcerations of the inguino-crural and buttocks folds. Indian J Dermatol 2011;56(1):101–3.
73. Preston PW, Hudson N, Lewis FM. Treatment of vulval Crohn's disease with infliximab. Clin Exp Dermatol 2006;31(3):378–80.
74. Rutgeerts P, Baert F. Immunosuppressive drugs in the treatment of Crohn's disease. Eur J Surg 1998;164:911–5.
75. Akintoye SO, Greenberg MS. Recurrent aphthous stomatitis. Dent Clin North Am 2014;58:281.
76. Hutton KP, Rogers RS 3rd. Recurrent aphthous stomatitis. Dermatol Clin 1987;5: 761–8.
77. Jorizzo JL, Taylor RS, Schmalstieg FC, et al. Complex aphthosis: a forme fruste of Behcet's syndrome. J Am Acad Dermatol 1985;13:80–4.
78. Schreiner DT, Jorizzo JL. Behcet's disease and complex aphthosis. Dermatol Clin 1987;5:769–78.
79. Ghate JV, Jorizzo JL. Behcet's disease and complex aphthosis. J Am Acad Dermatol 1999;40:1–18 [quiz: 19–20].
80. McCarty MA, Garton RA, Jorizzo JL. Complex aphthosis and Behcet's disease. Dermatol Clin 2003;21:41–8, vi.
81. Letsinger J, McCarty M, Jorizzo J. Complex aphthosis: a large case series with evaluation algorithm and therapeutic ladder from topicals to thalidomide. J Am Acad Dermatol 2005;52(3):500–8.
82. Lehman JS, Bruce AJ, Wetter DA, et al. Reactive nonsexually related acute genital ulcers: review of cases evaluated at Mayo clinic. J Am Acad Dermatol 2010; 63(1):44–51.
83. Gerber M, Deitch H, Mortensen J, et al. Vulvar ulcers in young females: a manifestation of aphthosis. J Pediatr Adolesc Gynecol 2006;19:195–204.
84. Farhi D, Wendling J, Molinari E, et al. Non–sexually related acute genital ulcers in 13 pubertal girls: a clinical and microbiological study. Arch Dermatol 2009; 145(1):38–45.
85. Criteria for diagnosis of Behçet's disease. International Study Group for Behçet's disease. Lancet 1990;335:1078.
86. Lynde C, Bruce A, Rogers R. Successful treatment of complex aphthosis with colchicine and dapsone. Arch Dermatol 2009;145(3):273–6.
87. Dixit S, Bradford J, Fischer G. Management of nonsexually acquired genital ulceration using oral and topical corticosteroids followed by doxycycline prophylaxis. J Am Acad Dermatol 2013;68:797–802.

Vulvovaginal Graft-Versus-Host Disease

Rachel I. Kornik, MD[a],*, Alison S. Rustagi, PhD[b]

KEYWORDS

- Graft-versus-host disease • Vulvovaginal • Genital
- Hematopoietic stem cell transplant

KEY POINTS

- Genital chronic graft-versus-host disease (cGVHD) is an underrecognized complication of hematopoietic stem cell transplantation (HCT) that has a significant impact on quality of life.
- Early diagnosis is essential to optimize treatment outcomes and avoid severe sequelae, such as anatomic disfigurement, sexual dysfunction, and pain.
- Patients should be educated on signs and symptoms of cGVHD and examined approximately 3 months after transplant to improve early detection.
- Treatment focuses on local immunosuppressive therapy with topical steroids, topical tacrolimus, and dilators to maintain vaginal patency. Addressing estrogen deficiency may be an important adjunct.
- Female recipients of allogeneic HCT are at higher risk of condylomas and cervical dysplasia and neoplasia. Performing cervical cytology screening may be prudent before and after HCT.

INTRODUCTION

There are approximately 8000 allogeneic hematopoietic stem cell transplants (HCT) performed in the United States each year, to treat a variety of malignant and nonmalignant conditions. This number has steadily increased over the past 3 decades and is likely to continue to increase,[1] requiring clinicians to become familiar with the issues facing this complex patient population.

PATHOPHYSIOLOGY

Chronic graft-versus-host disease (cGVHD) occurs when immunocompetent donor T cells recognize host tissue as foreign. This is a double-edged sword, because

Disclosure Statement: No disclosures to declare.
[a] Department of Dermatology, University of Wisconsin, 1 South Park Street, 7th Floor, Madison, WI 53715, USA; [b] UCSF School of Medicine, 505 Parnassus Avenue, San Francisco, CA 94143, USA
* Corresponding author.
E-mail address: rkornik@dermatology.wisc.edu

patients with cGVHD may have a reduced relapse rate, owing to graft-versus-tumor effect, but severe cGVHD has a profound effect on quality of life and mortality risk.[2,3] The pathophysiology of cGVHD is a complicated multi-step process. There is still much to be elucidated as current research points out. The sequence is likely triggered by the conditioning regimen which damages host tissue, particularly the gastrointestinal system, allowing the translocation of bacteria. The result is the release of cytokines and T-cell activation. The activated T-cells contribute to a pro-inflammatory cascade leading to dysregulation of both cell-mediated and humoral immunity. T-cell mediated toxicity and inflammation result in end-organ damage and fibrosis that is variable among patients.[4,5]

EPIDEMIOLOGY

GVHD is classified as acute or chronic based on clinical features rather than the temporal relationship to transplant.[6] Because there is very limited literature on acute GVHD affecting the genitals, this section focuses on cGVHD.

Chronic GVHD is the most common complication facing HCT patients with 60% to 70% affected at some point during their transplant course.[7,8] This number is increasing in frequency owing to a variety of factors: the increase in use of HCT, older recipient age, improvements in supportive care leading to increased survival, and more common use of peripheral blood stem cell grafts.[9,10] Chronic GVHD is the leading cause of nonrelapse mortality 2 years after transplantation. It also contributes to functional impairment, decreased mental health, and pain, resulting in a significant reduction in quality of life.[3,11]

The skin and mucous membranes are the most common sites of involvement followed by the liver and the eyes. Other less frequent sites include the gastrointestinal tract, lung, esophagus, female genital tract, male genitalia, and joints.[5,7]

The reported incidence of genital cGVHD varies according to study with a range of 19% to 52% of HCT recipients affected. Symptoms may be overlooked by patients and physicians alike, and are often misdiagnosed.[12,13] It has severe consequences for a woman's quality of life, including sexual health and interpersonal relationships, yet is rarely discussed before transplantation. Among 138 women who underwent allo-HCT at an institution in France that provided routine gynecologic follow-up at approximately 100 days after transplantation, 19% were diagnosed with genital cGVHD with a median follow-up time of 40 months (range, 13–117).[14] In a cohort of women (n = 61) undergoing active surveillance for genital cGVHD from 1999 to 2004, the cumulative incidence of genital cGVHD was 35% (95% CI, 25%–50%) and 49% (95% CI, 36%–63%) at 1 and 2 years, respectively, and was significantly higher among recipients of peripheral versus marrow blood progenitors (hazard ratio, 3.07; 95% CI, 1.22–7.73).[15] A retrospective study of 213 women from 1980 to 1999 found a cumulative genital cGVHD incidence of 25%.[16] In a cross-sectional study of 42 women evaluated at a median of 80 months posttransplantation (range, 13–148), 52% were diagnosed with genital cGVHD.[13] Reported median time of onset from transplant to genital cGVHD varies from 7[16] to 10[15,17] to 13 months,[14] but has been diagnosed up to 8 years after transplantation.[12,18] GVHD may manifest as GVHD prophylactic medications are tapered after transplantation, which varies from patient to patient.

Although risk factors for the development of chronic cGVHD are well-described and include a history of acute GVHD, older age of recipient, and a high degree of HLA mismatch,[9,10,19] risk factors for genital cGVHD are less well-characterized. Peripheral blood stem cell grafts correlate with increased risk of global cGVHD compared with bone marrow progenitors, a correlation that holds particularly true for genital manifestations of cGVHD.[15,20] The association between genital tract cGVHD with acute GVHD was assessed in 1 study of 32 patients with genital cGVHD and 50% of affected patients had a history of acute GVHD.[14] Neither parity nor positive vaginal culture (for streptococci, staphylococci, *Klebsiella, Proteus, Candida albicans,* etc) at the time of transplant seem to be associated with genital cGVHD risk,[16] although prior research found an association between genital tract infection and genital cGVHD risk.[21] In 1 study, donor sibling increased the risk of genital, but not extragenital, chronic GVHD compared with unrelated donor,[13] but this observation has not been corroborated elsewhere. Systemic corticosteroid use was associated with genital cGVHD in 1 study,[13] but this is likely due to confounding by indication, because cGVHD illness severity was not adjusted for and is strongly correlated with systemic steroid use. Exogenous estrogen therapy was borderline significantly associated with genital cGVHD in 1 study,[16] although unfortunately the authors did not specify the timing of estrogen therapy in relation to transplantation. The majority of women with genital cGVHD (73%–100%) show manifestations of extragenital cGVHD at the time of presentation,[12–14,16] most commonly the skin, mouth, and eyes.[12,14] Genital cGVHD can flare in synchrony with extragenital manifestations,[13] but may also persist despite good control of cGVHD in other systems. Presence of ocular and oral cGVHD increase the likelihood of involvement of other mucosal sites.[12,14,16] Importantly, there are reported cases of advanced genital cGVHD as the only or presenting manifestation of cGVHD.[14]

CLINICAL FEATURES

Genital cGVHD is often missed by the patient or her gynecologist owing to the nonspecific nature of presenting symptoms and low awareness of the condition.[12–14] As detailed, genital cGVHD usually presents in concert with other sites or systemic manifestations[12–14,16]; if it seems to be an isolated manifestation of cGVHD, other organ systems must be evaluated to rule out involvement. Dyspareunia, vaginal dryness or discharge, and vulvar pain are the most common presenting symptoms of genital GVHD (**Table 1**).[12,14] On examination, erythema and/or tenderness to palpation over Bartholin's or Skene's glands is consistent with genital cGVHD.[6,14] Skin changes include vulvar erythema, local mucosal paleness, and white/reticulated patches or plaques.[13,14] The disease favors the modified mucous membranes of the labia minora, perineum, clitoral prepuce, and vestibule while often sparing the fully keratinized labia majora. Genital cGVHD can visually seem identical to lichen sclerosus (**Fig. 1**) or lichen planus (**Fig. 2**). Lacy reticulations (Wickham striae) and erythematous patches with or without erosions and scarring are characteristic of lichen planus–like genital cGVHD, whereas lichen sclerosus–like genital cGVHD is more sclerotic, and characterized by hypopigmented, waxy-appearing, or hyperkeratotic plaques. Unlike idiopathic lichen sclerosus, lichen sclerosus–like genital cGVHD may be erosive and involve the mucosa. Vulvar fissures or erosions are found in approximately one-half of women at diagnosis (**Fig. 3**). Late complications of genital cGVHD include labial adhesions, clitoral agglutination, vaginal synechiae, circumferential fibrous banding, vaginal shortening, complete vaginal closure, and hematocolpos,[12,14,18,22–25] sometimes requiring surgical correction.[24,25] Vaginal synechiae are associated with sclerotic cGVHD of the skin ($P = .017$).[12,26] Vaginal fasciitis has also been reported in one patient with severe sclerotic GVHD.[12] Vulvar cGVHD typically precedes vaginal cGVHD,[12,16] with a median onset of vulvar GVHD of 9 months and a median onset of vaginal cGVHD of 19 months post-transplant.[12] Surveillance for vaginal cGVHD is

Table 1
Diagnosis and grading of genital chronic graft-versus-host disease—National Institutes of Health Guidelines

	Score 0	Score 1	Score 2	Score 3
Genital female	No signs	Mild signs and symptoms[a] with or without discomfort on examination[b] Any of following: Erythema on vulvar mucosal surfaces Vulvar lichen planus –like features[c] Vulvar lichen sclerosis–like features[c]	Moderate signs and may have symptoms with or without discomfort on examination[b] Any of following: Erosive inflammatory changes of the vulvar mucosa[d] Ulcers[d] Fissures in vulvar folds[d]	Severe signs with or without symptoms Any of following: Labial fusion[c] Clitoral hood agglutination[c] Vaginal scarring[c]: Fibrinous vaginal adhesions Circumferential Fibrous vaginal banding Vaginal shortening Synechia Dense sclerotic changes Complete vaginal stenosis

[a] Symptoms are not specific and can represent premature gonadal failure or infection.
[b] To be determined by specialist or trained medical provider; discomfort is defined as vulvar pain elicited by gentle touch with cotton swab to any of the following sites: vestibular glands, labia minora or majora.
[c] Diagnostic sign.
[d] Distinctive sign.
Adapted from Jagasia MH, Greinix HT, Arora M, et al. National Institutes of Health Consensus Development Project on criteria for clinical trials in chronic graft-versus-host disease: I. The 2014 Diagnosis and Staging Working Group Report. Biol Blood Marrow Transplant 2015;21(3):391–3; with permission.

important; detection at earlier stages has been shown to reduce the likelihood of surgical intervention.[15] Greater severity of disease at diagnosis is associated with a longer time from transplantation to gynecologic examination; in a French cohort, patients with grade I genital GVHD at diagnosis received a routine gynecology examination at a median of 111 days after transplantation, compared with 232 days for those diagnosed with grade III disease.[14] Together, these data highlight the importance of early recognition and treatment to prevent progression of disease. This may also support the inference that patients—even if symptomatic and/or those experiencing severe disease—may not present to a gynecologist in the absence of active surveillance. Moreover, the signs and symptoms of cGVHD overlap with other common vulvovaginal complaints, contributing to a delay in diagnosis. There are no reported cases of urethral involvement; however, given the involvement of other mucosal surfaces and similarity to lichen planus, which can involve the urethra,[27] urologic–gynecologic evaluation should be undertaken if a patient has urethral symptoms including burning or disruption of micturition. In sum, a high index of suspicion for genital GVHD is warranted for any woman with vulvovaginal and/or urinary symptoms and a history of allo-HCT.

Physical examination should include inspection of the vulva, with particular attention to the labia minora, prepuce, and introitus. A Q-tip may be used to gently assess for pain and/or burning on palpation of the vestibular glands, introitus, and labia minora and majora. Digital palpation of the vagina should be performed to assess for

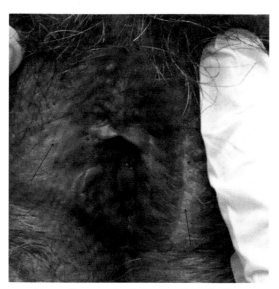

Fig. 1. Lichen sclerosus–like graft-versus-host disease (GVHD). There are subtle waxy hypo-pigmented patches of the interlabial sulci extending toward the anterior labial commissure (*arrows*). The labia minora are agglutinated (*arrow heads*). The clitoral prepuce is bound down. Lichen sclerosus–like GVHD and lichen sclerosis are challenging to distinguish, both clinically and histologically. In the post-hematopoietic stem cell transplantation setting these genital findings are considered diagnostic of chronic GVHD. (*From* Curtis L, Kornik RI, Mays JW, et al. Clinical presentation of mucosal acute and chronic graft-versus-host disease. In: Cotliar JA, editor. Atlas of graft-versus-host disease: approaches to diagnosis and treatment. Springer International Publishing AG; 2017. p. 35; with permission of Springer.)

synechiae, narrowing, shortening, or other signs of scarring.[28] Visual examination of the vagina via a speculum examination may also be helpful to assess for vaginal erosions, ulceration, or erythema, but may not be possible if scarring is advanced or the patient is in pain. Saline wet mount may be used to assess for vaginal inflammation and infection; the presence of parabasilar cells, lack of lactobacilli, and increase in proportion of white blood cells to squamous cells is suggestive of vaginal cGVHD, but may also be seen in atrophic vaginitis. However, atrophic vaginitis should resolve with intravaginal estrogen alone, unlike cGVHD which also requires local immunosuppression. Serial wet mounts, in addition to a digital examination and visual inspection, may be used to monitor the response to the treatment. It is especially helpful if a speculum examination cannot be performed. A decrease in inflammatory cells, return of lactobacilli, and normalization of squamous cells are signs of a healthy vaginal mucosa. Although there is no data on perianal involvement, the entire anogenital region may be involved and should be examined as well.

DIAGNOSTIC CRITERIA

The 2014 National Institutes of Health Diagnosis and Staging Working Group Report defined diagnostic and distinctive signs and grading criteria (see **Table 1**).[6] These criteria were updated in 2014 to emphasize that severity of disease is not solely dependent on patient-reported symptoms or discomfort with examination. Diagnostic signs are sufficient to establish the diagnosis of cGVHD without further investigation.

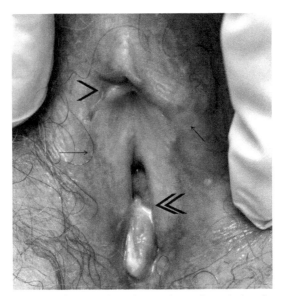

Fig. 2. Lichen planus–like graft-versus-host disease (GVHD). Reticulate leucokeratosis (Wickham striae) with erythematous patches mimic lichen planus (*small arrows*). There is scarring with complete resorption of labia minora, clitoral hood agglutination, and narrowing of the vaginal orifice (*large arrow heads*). This patient displays severe signs of GVHD. Scarring is irreversible and vaginal stenosis, synechiae, and adhesions require surgical correction to maintain sexual function. There is incidental vaginal prolapse in this photo. (*From* Curtis L, Kornik RI, Mays JW, et al. Clinical presentation of mucosal acute and chronic graft-versus-host disease. In: Cotliar JA, editor. Atlas of graft-versus-host disease: approaches to diagnosis and treatment. Springer International Publishing AG; 2017. p. 35; with permission of Springer.)

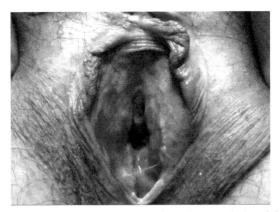

Fig. 3. Erosive graft-versus-host disease (GVHD). The vulvar vestibule exhibits erythematous patches and erosions extending toward the vaginal mucosa. There is a thin white plaque at the posterior fourchette. There is subtle fusion of the labia minora. (*From* Curtis L, Kornik RI, Mays JW, et al. Clinical presentation of mucosal acute and chronic graft-versus-host disease. In: Cotliar JA, editor. Atlas of graft-versus-host disease: approaches to diagnosis and treatment. Springer International Publishing AG; 2017. p. 35; with permission of Springer.)

Distinctive signs require additional testing, such as a biopsy or diagnostic features at another site. The unequivocal diagnosis of chronic GVHD requires at least 1 diagnostic manifestation of chronic GVHD or at least 1 distinctive manifestation plus a pertinent biopsy, laboratory finding, or evaluation by a specialist.

Biopsy and Histology

The National Institutes of Health 2014 Consensus Conference on the histopathologic diagnosis of cGVHD provides updated guidelines on the interpretation and use of biopsies in the diagnosis and management of patients with cGVHD. The report reminds the reader that biopsies are a "snapshot in time of a complex and dynamic biological process that reflects the duration, use of immunosuppressive therapy, the possibility of more than one process, the location and the quality of the sample."[28] Rather than a test, a biopsy should be considered as consultation with the interpreting pathologist. The addition of clinical context is essential to arrive at the correct diagnosis. All biopsy reports should include pertinent information about the patient's transplant history and description of clinical signs, morphology of the lesion(s), distribution and arrangement, duration, and current and past treatments.[29] A biopsy is particularly helpful in establishing the diagnosis of cGVHD of the genital tract if there are no diagnostic clinical findings,[13] if the presentation is atypical, or if other differential diagnoses such as infection or dysplasia/cancer are in consideration.[28] Choosing the right location and timing of a biopsy is important to obtain a successful sample. If completed early on before the development of well-established lesions, the findings may be subtle or nonspecific.[12] Similar to other erosive conditions of the vulva, a biopsy of the center of an erosion or ulcer rather than the border with intact skin will often yield nonspecific results. Chronic GVHD may be suppressed by systemic or topical immunosuppressive therapies, and ideally a sample should be obtained from untreated skin or mucosa. If it is not possible to disrupt therapy, the pathologist should be made aware of current treatments that may blunt the inflammatory response. Certain body locations may be more technically challenging to biopsy, leading to inadequate sampling, sheared tissues, or crush artifact. Improper tissue processing or sectioning can miss key histologic features.[28] Finally, a biopsy to confirm cGVHD may be deferred if a patient is in significant pain.[30] The application of a topical anesthetic prior to injection of intradermal anesthesia will often increase the tolerability of a biopsy. A 4-mm full-thickness punch biopsy is usually sufficient to obtain an adequate sample. For thin or very small samples, the authors find that placing the specimen skin side up on a firm piece of paper before submerging in formalin can help with orienting and processing of the specimen. Interpretation by a pathologist or dermatopathologist with experience in reading skin and mucous membrane inflammatory conditions may also be helpful.

The histology of cGVHD of the vulvar and vaginal area is similar to that described in the skin and oral mucosa.[28] Spiryda and colleagues[17] reported the histopathology of 7 biopsy specimens from patients with vaginal cGVHD. One patient's specimen demonstrated lichenoid dermatitis, whereas the others showed foci of inflammation, hyperkeratosis, and spongiosis. Knutsson and colleagues evaluated biopsy specimens of 38 women after HCT using histologic grading criteria defined by Shulman and colleagues.[30] Of 14 patients with diagnostic clinical signs, 6 had either no cGVHD or possible cGVHD by histologic grade. Conversely, of 24 patients with no diagnostic clinical signs of genital cGVHD, 7 had histologic features that were consistent with cGVHD, thereby highlighting the challenges in obtaining a histopathologic diagnosis and the need for additional clinical context. The vulvar mucosa often has a background of nonspecific chronic inflammation complicating the picture further.[31,32]

Specific criteria for cGVHD outlined in the 2014 NIH Consensus Development Project on Criteria for Clinical Trials in Chronic Graft-versus-Host Disease GVHD pathology working group include lichen planus–like changes (combination of epidermal thickening, hypergranulosis and acanthosis with bandlike infiltrate of lymphocytes along the dermal–epidermal junction, and blunted rete ridges) and lichen sclerosis–like changes. Vacuolar change centered around eccrine coils is highly specific for GVHD. However, the labia minora, vestibule, and vaginal mucosa (ie, the areas commonly involved in genital cGVHD) are devoid of eccrine glands.[29,33] Lichenoid cGVHD is histomorphologically indistinguishable from idiopathic or drug-induced planus and the clinical context may be necessary for the pathologist to arrive at the correct diagnosis.[33] Lichen sclerosus–like findings include homogenization of dermal collagen, overlying interface change, and sparse lymphocytic infiltrations[28] (**Fig. 4**). Sclerotic cGVHD histologically mimics idiopathic lichen sclerosus.

DIFFERENTIAL DIAGNOSES

The varied clinical manifestations of cGVHD create a broad differential. Symptoms of vulvar and/or vaginal cGVHD such as burning, pruritis, dyspareunia, and vaginal dryness overlap with estrogen deficiency.[16,17] Treatment with topical estrogen will improve symptoms of local estrogen deficiency but will not be sufficient to treat cGVHD.[16] Systematic assessment for all potential differential diagnosis is especially relevant on the vulvar skin, which is prone to irritant dermatitis, atrophic vaginitis, and common infections such as candida, human papillomavirus (HPV), and herpes simplex virus. Dyspareunia and introital burning may also mimic vulvodynia, which is a diagnosis of exclusion.[12,14,16] Immunosuppressed patients have an increased risk of secondary malignancy and require monitoring for vulvar intraepithelial neoplasia and squamous cell carcinoma, which can present as an erythematous patch, erosion/ulcer, verrucous lesion, or dyspigmentation.[34] It is not uncommon for patients with cGVHD to present with a concomitant diagnosis or develop additional issues over their course, necessitating frequent reevaluation of symptoms, particularly if a patient is not responding as expected to treatment. Lichen planus and lichen sclerosus are the 2 most likely inflammatory diagnoses to be considered in the differential diagnosis of

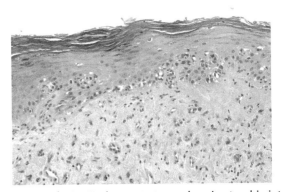

Fig. 4. This vulvar biopsy of cGVHD demonstrates a chronic atrophic interface dermatitis with muted rete ridges, scattered perijunctional necrotic keratinocytes, slight hypergranulosis, and hyperkeratosis. There is also slight sclerosis of the subepithelial tissue with associated neovascularization. All of these characteristics are common to lichen sclerosus. (*Courtesy of* T. McCalmont, MD, San Francisco, CA.)

cGVHD. However, these clinical findings are diagnostic of cGVHD in the right context. **Table 2** summarizes the differential diagnosis of cGVHD and suggested evaluation.

MANAGEMENT OF CHRONIC GRAFT-VERSUS-HOST DISEASE

Early diagnosis of vulvovaginal cGVHD, before significant scarring, allows for the greatest likelihood of successful treatment and resolution of the disease.[14,15] Management of cGVHD of the genital area often requires a multidisciplinary approach and collaboration with a genital specialist or provider with experience in the management of genital/mucosal cGVHD. Unfortunately, there are no randomized, controlled trials investigating the treatment of vulvovaginal cGVHD and optimal therapy is tailored to the individual based on the severity and location of involvement. The treatment is similar to other scarring or erosive mucosal diseases, such as lichen planus and lichen sclerosus. The main treatments are topical and include immunosuppressive therapies and estrogens.[12,15,17] Although there are no studies on systemic immunosuppression for the treatment of genital disease alone, severe or recalcitrant cases may not respond adequately to topical therapies[17]. Co-management with the transplant team/hematologist is necessary when systemic therapies are considered in addition to topical treatments.

First-line treatment of vulvar cGVHD is with a high-potency topical steroid, such as clobetasol proprionate ointment (0.05%) applied once to twice daily depending on severity. An ointment base is preferable to a cream, because it has increased permeability, emollient effect, and is less likely to contain preservatives, which can cause irritation.[32] The clinician should demonstrate to the patient where and how to apply a thin film of the medication to avoid atrophy of nonaffected areas. Response to treatment is assessed at 4-6 week intervals for patients with moderated to severe disease, sooner for worsening symptoms. The interval may increased to 8-12 weeks for patients with well-controlled or mild disease. If clinical signs and symptoms improve, the application may be tapered to a maintenance regimen of 2 to 3 times a week.[6,15] If response to a topical steroid alone is inadequate, topical tacrolimus (0.1%) ointment may be prescribed alone or in conjunction with topical steroids. It can cause significant stinging and burning, especially when applied to inflamed or nonintact mucosa. If patients are able to tolerate the burning, it often subsides with continued application and may be mitigated by an initial period of topical steroid use.[35]

Treating vaginal involvement requires some resourcefulness due to the lack of commercially available vaginal steroid preparations. Hydrocortisone acetate rectal suppositories (25 mg) are commercially available but may not be potent enough to treat severe disease. Hydrocortisone acetate (10%) is available as a rectal foam or may be compounded into a gentle base suitable for mucosa, then inserted into the vagina using a vaginal applicator. Intravaginal clindamycin 2% may be added to a steroid base for additional antiinflammatory effect. One proposed regimen is hydrocortisone 10% in 2% clindamycin base: apply 5 g with vaginal applicator every other night for 4 weeks and then assess for response.[6] Other alternatives include specially compounded tacrolimus suppository (2 mg tacrolimus per 2 g suppository), cyclosporine, or steroid creams and suppositories (**Table 3**). The cost of specially compounded medications may be prohibitive. A pea-sized amount of clobetasol or tacrolimus ointment (with or without estrogen) may be placed at the tip of a dilator and inserted into the vagina approximately 3 times a week as well.[12,26] Treatment should be tapered to the lowest medication frequency and concentration that controls disease. Patients may require a maintenance therapy to prevent relapse.[15,17] If therapy is stopped because of adequate response, patients should be monitored for relapse, which may not be symptomatic. Interested readers are also pointed to supplement 5 of the 2014 NIH

Table 2
Differential diagnosis of genital GVHD by clinical features

	Vulvovaginal Dryness	Vulvovaginal Erosions and Ulcerations	Mucosal Erythema	White Patches and Plaques	Vulvar Pain and/or Dyspareunia	Vaginal Discharge
DDx	Estrogen deficiency Drug induced[a]	Viral infection[b] Secondary malignancy Candidiasis Bacterial infection Sexually transmitted infections[c] Drug reaction[d]	Estrogen deficiency Erythematous candidiasis Bacterial infection Irritant or allergic contact dermatitis VIN Plasma cell mucositis	Lichen planus[e] Lichen sclerosus[e] Lichen simplex chronicus Vitiligo Postinflammatory pigment alteration Candidiasis Condyloma VIN/squamous cell carcinoma	Estrogen deficiency Vulvodynia[e]	Candidiasis Bacterial infection[f] Trichomoniasis Atrophic vaginitis Vaginal intraepithelial neoplasia Vaginal condyloma Cervicitis[g] Foreign body Irritant or allergic contact dermatitis
Useful tests	Consider trial of topical/intravaginal estrogen if no contraindications Consider skin biopsy to assess for features of GVHD	Viral direct fluorescent antibody, PCR and/or culture KOH preparation and fungal culture Bacterial culture STD testing as appropriate Diagnostic biopsy of affected, intact skin adjacent to defect	Assess for irritants[h] KOH preparation and fungal culture for Candida Bacterial culture Diagnostic skin biopsy	KOH preparation and fungal culture for Candida Diagnostic skin biopsy	Consider trial of topical/intravaginal estrogen if no contraindications Consider skin biopsy to assess for features of GVHD	Saline wet mount KOH preparation and fungal culture for Candida Amine whiff test Vaginal pH Consider bacterial culture Consider vaginal biopsy

Abbreviations: DDx, differential diagnosis; GVHD, graft-versus-host disease; KOH, potassium hydroxide; PCR, polymerase chain reaction; STD, sexually transmitted disease; VIN, vulvar intraepithelial neoplasia.

[a] Main culprit medications with antiestrogen effect: tamoxifen, medroxyprogesterone, and aromatase inhibitors.

[b] Herpes simplex, herpes zoster, cytomegalovirus, Epstein-Barr virus, and human immunodeficiency virus (HIV).

[c] Syphilis and HIV.

[d] Fixed drug eruption, Stevens-Johnson syndrome, and toxic epidermal necrolysis.

[e] Only if present before transplantation.

[f] Bacterial vaginosis, and Staphylococcus aureus, group A Streptococcus.

[g] Gonorrhea, chlamydia, herpes simplex virus, and trichomonas.

[h] Personal care products, topical prescription preparations, urine, and feces.

From Curtis L, Kornik RI, Mays JW, et al. Clinical presentation of mucosal acute and chronic graft-versus-host disease: approaches to diagnosis and treatment. Springer International Publishing AG; 2017. p. 29–42; with permission of Springer.

Table 3
Chronic GVHD: Topical therapies[a], supportive measures and monitoring

Treatment	Lichen sclerosus/lichen planus–like changes or erosions involving the vulva
	Consider referral to a specialist
	Correction of estrogen deficiency with topical estrogen if no contraindications, *plus*:
	High-potency topical steroid ointment
	Tacrolimus ointment 0.1% alone or in addition to a topical steroid
	Female genital lichen planus–like changes or erosions also involving vaginal mucosa
	As above *plus:*
	Intravaginal estrogen if no contraindication
	Intravaginal steroid (using applicator, dilator or suppository)
	Tacrolimus cream/suppository 0.1% (2 mg tacrolimus per 2 g suppository)[b]
	Dilator therapy
	Vaginal stenosis/synechiae (fibrosis):
	As above, *plus*
	Surgical intervention for lysis of adhesions or vaginal reconstruction as necessary
	Dilator therapy to prevent recurrence
Preventative/ supportive measures	Surveillance for estrogen deficiency
	Education for patients on signs and symptoms of cGVHD
	Intermittent dilator use for non–sexually active patients
	Vulvar hygiene to minimize irritation
	Use of nonirritating personal lubricants
	Simple emollient to the vulva
	Surveillance for infection and secondary malignancy
Recommended monitoring	Genital examination, including inspection of vulva, vaginal mucosa, and cervix at 3–6 mo after transplantation or sooner based on symptoms, then at least annually
	Consider gynecologic examination at a minimum of every 3 mo for patients with known active genital chronic GVHD
	Cervical cytology testing annually or more frequently based on results
	Consider HPV vaccination
	Flare: rule out infection and allergic or irritant contact dermatitis

Abbreviations: GVHD, graft-versus-host disease; HPV, human papillomavirus.

[a] Topical therapy is most effective for GVHD involving isolated mucosal sites or for GVHD of isolated sites that is recalcitrant to systemic therapy. Topical therapies may need to be used in combination with systemic agents for management of severe localized GVHD or multiorgan involvement of GVHD.

[b] Intravaginal preparations may need to be specially compounded, and patients should be monitored for systemic absorption.

From Curtis L, Kornik RI, Mays JW, et al. Clinical presentation of mucosal acute and chronic graft-versus-host disease. In: Cotliar JA, editor. Atlas of graft-versus-host disease: approaches to diagnosis and treatment. Springer International Publishing AG; 2017. p. 29–42; with permission of Springer.

recommendations for ancillary and supportive care, which outlines different treatment regimens. Dilators are a crucial part of detecting disease in non–sexually active patients as well as treating and preventing, scarring, narrowing, and shortening of the vagina. Dilator therapy should be instituted early if there are signs of vaginal involvement including erosions/ulcers or scarring. If vaginal scarring presents as filamentous strands, they may be separated with a finger during vaginal examination.[12] Surgery may be necessary for severe vulvar[36] and vaginal scarring to restore sexual function and to access the cervix if cytologic monitoring is required.[12,15–17,37] Rarely, urgent surgery may be required if scarring impairs micturition.[36]

IATROGENIC EFFECTS AND POTENTIAL COMPLICATIONS

Patients using chronic topical steroids should be monitored for common adverse reactions. Steroid treatment can lead to reversible atrophy of the skin, manifested by telangiectasia and/or striae.[38] Topical estrogen may mitigate some of these side effects by promoting the thickness of vulvar epithelium.[12] Atrophy is somewhat less of a concern on the modified mucous membranes of the vulva and the mucosa, which are relatively resistant to thinning.[39] Rarely, topical steroids cause irritation or burning. Patients may also develop an allergic contact dermatitis to a vehicle or the steroid itself. Clobetasol preparations often contains propylene glycol, a well-known skin irritant[40]; if the patient experiences a burning sensation with application that does not resolve, an alternative high-potency topical steroid without propylene glycol or tacrolimus ointment may be tried. If topical steroids are discontinued abruptly, a rebound flare or withdrawal may be precipitated. Withdrawal symptoms are characterized by burning/stinging sensation, pruritus, and pain, erythema, pustules, edema, and dryness/friability, starting 14 to 21 days after steroid cessation.[41] However, most cases were reported after prolonged, inappropriate use of high-potency steroids. Topical immunosuppression increases the likelihood of superficial infections such as candida, bacteria, HPV, and herpes outbreaks. Patients should be monitored for infections routinely, particularly if symptoms worsen or flare while on therapy. The severe consequences of untreated genital cGVHD far outweigh these risks, but monitoring for adverse effects should nonetheless be a component of ongoing follow-up. If long-term use of high-potency intravaginal steroids or tacrolimus is anticipated, providers should be aware of the risk of systemic absorption. Although there is no data on systemic absorption from intravaginal use of these agents in the literature, there is evidence of absorption from the oral mucosa,[42,43] which has similar histology and permeability.[44] If prolonged use of intravaginal tacrolimus and/or steroids is considered, after the monitoring parameters for the systemic use of these medications is prudent.

SUPPORTIVE CARE

The National Institutes of Health consensus project has published guidelines for ancillary therapy and supportive care of vulvar and vaginal cGVHD.[32] As transplant patients live longer, providing ancillary and supportive care, which includes education, preventative care, and treatment, has become essential to the well-being of the patient.

The role of general skin care and topical estrogen is highlighted in the guidelines, although evidence is anecdotal. Almost all women undergoing transplant in their reproductive years experience ovarian failure due to the conditioning regimen.[45] Addressing estrogen deficiency after HCT is important as an adjuvant in treatment of vulvovaginal cGVHD.[26,46] Without sufficient estrogen, the vulvar and vaginal epithelium becomes thin, fragile, and more susceptible to irritation and trauma. Estrogen is also thought to have a role in maintaining the optimal vaginal pH. In well-estrogenized tissue, mature, glycogen-rich cells shed and act as a substrate for lactobacilli, which create lactic acid.[47] When lactic acid is reduced, the vaginal pH increases, contributing to dysbiosis, which in turn contributes to vaginal inflammation and increased risk of vaginal infection.[48] The microbiota of the vagina and its relationship to infection, inflammation, and GVHD is an area that requires further investigation.[46] The addition of estrogen may improve the integrity and barrier function of the vulvar and vaginal epithelium and help to restore microbial homeostasis.[49] Although estrogen by itself is not a treatment for cGVHD,[17] it eliminates concomitant estrogen deficiency to improve tissue resiliency and helps to mitigate the effect of treatments such as steroid atrophy and improve symptoms.[12,26] Topical/local estrogen is preferred as a treatment for skin and mucosal symptoms because of its effectiveness and safety compared with systemic estrogen. However, patients on systemic estrogen for other ovarian failure symptoms may still benefit from additional low-dose local therapy.[46,50] Estrogen therapy in any form should be initiated in conjunction with a gynecologist or physician with experience in the management of ovarian failure. Although topical preparations are considered safe, there is still a limited amount of systemic absorption, especially across inflamed mucosa, that may be contraindicated in certain patient populations (history of an estrogen-sensitive tumor, thrombosis, liver disease, etc).[51] Although the risk of endometrial cancer is thought to be of little concern for low-dose topical estrogen, safety has not been studied past 1 year.[51] The lowest dose preparation should be used to control symptoms. A frequently recommended course of treatment is daily application to the vulva for 2 weeks then decrease to 2 to 3 times a week. There are multiple vaginal preparations that can be used in a similar fashion. The estradiol vaginal ring helps to treat dyspareunia and may mechanically prevent vaginal stenosis,[12] although caution should be used if there are mucosal erosions or ulcerations because the mechanical pressure can aggravate tissues and scarring has been reported to occur below the ring.[12]

If estrogen is contraindicated, the patient may benefit from the use of a vaginal moisturizer such as Replens.[51] A discussion of nonhormonal treatments of vulvovaginal atrophy is beyond the scope of this article, but it would be interesting to investigate their potential as an adjuvant treatment in genital cGVHD.

As with any inflammatory vulvovaginal condition, patients should also be informed of the importance of gentle genital care to improve barrier function and avoid irritants. Soap, fragrances, feminine washes or wipes, and daily use of pantiliners should be avoided.[32,39] A daily emollient such as petrolatum is recommended after bathing, as are silicone- or water-based lubricants for sexual activity.

PREVENTION AND SURVEILLANCE

Systematic surveillance for genital cGVHD should be included in the long-term management of all female allo-HCT recipients.[14,26] It is common for women to misattribute symptoms or be too embarrassed to bring up personal issues related to their genitalia or sexuality.[52,53] Therefore, all women should be questioned about sexual issues, urinary symptoms, and other symptoms of vulvovaginal cGVHD at routine follow-up and educated on how to perform a self-examine. According to the National Institutes of Health Ancillary and Supportive Care Working Group Report, gynecologic evaluation is recommended before HCT and beginning 100 days after HCT to identify cGVHD early and initiate management. It is equally important to include patient education about sexual and gynecologic dysfunctions common after HCT so that patients are involved in self-monitoring. If patients are not sexually active, they may use a dilator to check vaginal patency within 3 months of transplantation.[32] In addition, the recognition of cutaneous or mucosal GVHD should prompt a gynecologic examination owing to their high cooccurrence of genital cGVHD, even if the patient does not endorse genital symptoms.[14,26,46] The specific frequency of examinations depends on age, pretransplant Pap smear frequency, history of abnormal Pap smears, and other patient factors, but such follow-up should include a minimum of annual pelvic examinations for patients without genital cGVHD, and referral to a gynecologist or provider with experience in inflammatory genital conditions for any vulvovaginal symptoms. In women with known genital cGVHD or severe extragenital cGVHD, a pelvic examination performed every 3 months or less is the standard of care to monitor for progression of disease, treatment, and response.[26]

Female recipients of allo-HCT are at higher risk of condylomas and cervical dysplasia and neoplasia; cervical cancer incidence is up to 13 times higher among this group compared with the general population.[54] This pattern is likely due to systemic immunosuppression and resulting reactivation of HPV, because a longer duration of immunosuppressive therapy is associated with higher incidence of genital HPV disease,[55] and is also observed in recipients of solid organ transplants and in patients with HIV.[56] In the French cohort, 8 of 32 patients (25%) developed condylomas during follow-up, and 1 of 32 (3%) developed cervical dysplasia.[14] In a cohort of 35 women who underwent cervical cytology testing after allo-HCT, 43% of women had abnormal results; in a subgroup analysis, genital cGVHD was not associated with abnormal Pap smear results, although immunosuppression to manage chronic cGVHD was associated with abnormal cervical cytology (adjusted odds ratio, 4.6; 95% CI, 1.1–16.4).[55] In a more recent case report, local immunosuppressive therapy to treat genital cGVHD was associated with rapid condyloma development.[57] Consequently, it may be prudent to consider collecting cervical cytology and HPV DNA tests before initiating therapy for genital cGVHD.[57] HPV vaccination could theoretically prevent cervical dysplasia,[58] although the blunted immune response in the setting of immunosuppression may limit vaccination efficacy. Pretransplantation HPV testing could stratify women by risk of developing subsequent genital HPV disease. The actual efficacies of these approaches are unknown,[55,58] although this is an area of active investigation and a phase I randomized controlled trial is currently testing the efficacy of posttransplantation HPV vaccination (ClinicalTrials.gov identifier: NCT01092195).

Currently, based on expert opinion, annual cytology is standard of care for all women after allo-HCT, with reflex high-risk HPV DNA testing for normal or atypical squamous cells of undetermined significance cytology results, or colposcopy for atypical squamous cells cannot rule out high-grade dysplasia or worse.[26] It has been proposed that patients should be evaluated for HPV disease before initiating topical immunosuppression.[26] The management of genital cGVHD with immunosuppression in the setting of cervical or vulvar dysplasia is complex and requires a multidisciplinary approach that is tailored to the individual.

SUMMARY

Genital cGVHD is a common complication of allo-HCT that can dramatically affect quality of life and interpersonal relationships, and is a common cause of vulvovaginal symptoms in female recipients of allo-HCT. Fortunately, the astute clinician can detect genital cGVHD early. With a thorough history, physical examination, and if necessary, biopsy, the most morbid complications can be prevented with available, effective treatment options. Patient education is also important to empower women to seek care early. Although often challenging, caring for women after HCT offers the provider an opportunity to have a meaningful impact on patient's lives.

REFERENCES

1. Pasquini MC, Zhu X. Current uses and outcomes of hematopoietic stem cell transplantation: CIBMTR summary slides, 2015. Available at: http://www.cibmtr.org. Accessed January 10, 2017.

2. Inamoto Y, Martin PJ, Storer BE, et al. Association of severity of organ involvement with mortality and recurrent malignancy in patients with chronic graft-versus-host disease. Haematologica 2014;99:1618–23.

3. Lee SJ, Kim HT, Ho VT, et al. Quality of life associated with acute and chronic graft-versus-host disease. Bone Marrow Transplant 2006;38:305–10.

4. Zhang L, Chu J, Yu J, et al. Cellular and molecular mechanisms in graft-versus-host disease. J Leukoc Biol 2016;99:279–87.

5. Flowers MED, Martin PJ. How we treat chronic graft-versus-host disease. Blood 2015;125:606–15.

6. Carpenter PA, Kitko CL, Elad S, et al. National Institutes of Health Consensus Development Project on Criteria for Clinical Trials in Chronic Graft-versus-Host Disease: V. The 2014 Ancillary Therapy and Supportive Care Working Group Report. Biol Blood Marrow Transplant 2015;21(7):1167–87.

7. Lee SJ. Severity of chronic graft-versus-host disease: association with treatment-related mortality and relapse. Blood 2002;100:406–14.

8. Lee SJ, Vogelsang G, Flowers MED. Chronic graft-versus-host disease. Biol Blood Marrow Transplant 2003;9:215–33.

9. Hymes SR, Alousi AM, Cowen EW. Graft-versus-host disease: part I. Pathogenesis and clinical manifestations of graft-versus-host disease. J Am Acad Dermatol 2012;66:515.e1-18 [quiz: 533–4].

10. Arai S, Arora M, Wang T, et al. Increasing incidence of chronic graft-versus-host disease in allogeneic transplantation: a report from the Center for International Blood and Marrow Transplant Research. Biol Blood Marrow Transplant 2015;21: 266–74.

11. Baker KS, Fraser CJ. Quality of life and recovery after graft-versus-host disease. Best Pract Res Clin Haematol 2008;21:333–41.

12. Stratton P, Turner ML, Childs R, et al. Vulvovaginal chronic graft-versus-host disease with allogeneic hematopoietic stem cell transplantation. Obstet Gynecol 2007;110:1041–9.

13. Smith Knutsson E, Björk Y, Broman AK, et al. Genital chronic graft-versus-host disease in females: a cross-sectional study. Biol Blood Marrow Transplant 2014;20:806–11.

14. Hirsch P, Leclerc M, Rybojad M, et al. Female genital chronic graft-versus-host disease: importance of early diagnosis to avoid severe complications. Transplantation 2012;93:1265–9.

15. Zantomio D, Grigg AP, MacGregor L, et al. Female genital tract graft-versus-host disease: incidence, risk factors and recommendations for management. Bone Marrow Transplant 2006;38:567–72.

16. Spinelli S, Chiodi S, Costantini S, et al. Female genital tract graft-versus-host disease following allogeneic bone marrow transplantation. Haematologica 2003;88: 1163–8.

17. Spiryda LB, Laufer MR, Soiffer RJ, et al. Graft-versus-host disease of the vulva and/or vagina: diagnosis and treatment. Biol Blood Marrow Transplant 2003;9: 760–5.

18. Riera C, Deroover Y, Marechal M. Severe vaginal chronic graft-versus-host disease (GVHD): two cases with late onset and literature review. Eur J Gynaecol Oncol 2010;31:703–4.

19. Lee SJ, Vogelsang G, Gilman A, et al. A survey of diagnosis, management, and grading of chronic GVHD. Biol Blood Marrow Transplant 2002;8:32–9.

20. Flowers MED. Comparison of chronic graft-versus-host disease after transplantation of peripheral blood stem cells versus bone marrow in allogeneic recipients: long-term follow-up of a randomized trial. Blood 2002;100:415–9.

21. Bradbury C. Clinical bone marrow transplantation: a reference textbook. New York: Cambridge University Press; 1994.

22. DeLord C, Treleaven J, Shepherd J, et al. Vaginal stenosis following allogeneic bone marrow transplantation for acute myeloid leukaemia. Bone Marrow Transplant 1999;23:523–5.

23. Anguenot JL, Ibéchéole V, Helg C, et al. Vaginal stenosis with hematocolpometra, complicating chronic graft versus host disease. Eur J Obstet Gynecol Reprod Biol 2002;103:185–7.

24. Costantini S, Di Capua E, Bosi S, et al. The management of severe vaginal obstruction from genital chronic graft-versus-host disease: diagnosis, surgical technique and follow-up. Minerva Ginecol 2006;58:11–6.

25. Norian JM, Stratton P. Labial fusion: a rare complication of chronic graft-versus-host disease. Obstet Gynecol 2008;112:437–9.

26. Shanis D, Merideth M, Pulanic TK, et al. Female long-term survivors after allogeneic hematopoietic stem cell transplantation: evaluation and management. Semin Hematol 2012;49:83–93.

27. Verma P, Pandhi D. Lichen planus of the external urinary meatus masquerading sexually transmitted disease. Int J STD AIDS 2012;23:73–4.

28. Shulman HM, Cardona DM, Greenson JK, et al. NIH consensus development project on criteria for clinical trials in chronic graft-versus-host disease: II. The 2014 Pathology Working Group Report. Biol Blood Marrow Transplant 2015;21: 589–603.

29. Hillen U, Häusermann P, Massi D, et al. Consensus on performing skin biopsies, laboratory workup, evaluation of tissue samples and reporting of the results in patients with suspected cutaneous graft-versus-host disease. J Eur Acad Dermatol Venereol 2015;29:948–54.

30. Shulman HM, Kleiner D, Lee SJ, et al. Histopathologic diagnosis of chronic graft-versus-host disease: National Institutes of Health Consensus Development Project on Criteria for Clinical Trials in Chronic Graft-versus-Host Disease: II. Pathology Working Group Report. Biol Blood Marrow Transplant 2006;12:31–47.

31. Lundqvist EN, Hofer PA, Olofsson JI, et al. Is vulvar vestibulitis an inflammatory condition? A comparison of histological findings in affected and healthy women. Acta Derm Venereol 1997;77:319–22.

32. Carpenter PA, Kitko CL, Elad S, et al. National Institutes of Health Consensus Development Project on criteria for clinical trials in chronic graft-versus-host disease: V. The 2014 Ancillary Therapy and Supportive Care Working Group Report. Biol Blood Marrow Transplant 2015;21:1167–87.

33. Ziemer M. Graft-versus-host disease of the skin and adjacent mucous membranes: graft-versus-host disease of the skin. J Dtsch Dermatol Ges 2013;11: 477–95.

34. Léonard B, Kridelka F, Delbecque K, et al. A clinical and pathological overview of vulvar condyloma acuminatum, intraepithelial neoplasia, and squamous cell carcinoma. Biomed Res Int 2014;2014:1–11.

35. Frankel HC, Qureshi AA. Comparative effectiveness of topical calcineurin inhibitors in adult patients with atopic dermatitis. Am J Clin Dermatol 2012;13:113–23.

36. Scrivani C, Merideth MA, Klepac Pulanic T, et al. Early diagnosis of labial fusion in women after allogeneic hematopoietic cell transplant enables outpatient treatment. J Low Genit Tract Dis 2017;21(2):157–60.

37. Costantini S, Chiodi S, Spinelli S, et al. Complete vaginal obstruction caused by chronic graft- *versus* -host disease after haematopoietic stem cell transplantation: diagnosis and treatment. J Obstet Gynaecol 2004;24:591–5.
38. Katz HI, Prawer SE, Mooney JJ, et al. Preatrophy: covert sign of thinned skin. J Am Acad Dermatol 1989;20:731–5.
39. Thorstensen KA, Birenbaum DL. Recognition and management of vulvar dermatologic conditions: lichen sclerosus, lichen planus, and lichen simplex chronicus. J Midwifery Womens Health 2012;57:260–75.
40. Lessmann H, Schnuch A, Geier J, et al. Skin-sensitizing and irritant properties of propylene glycol. Contact Dermatitis 2005;53:247–59.
41. Hajar T, Leshem YA, Hanifin JM, et al. A systematic review of topical corticosteroid withdrawal ('steroid addiction') in patients with atopic dermatitis and other dermatoses. J Am Acad Dermatol 2015;72:541–9.e2.
42. Varoni EM, Molteni A, Sardella A, et al. Pharmacokinetics study about topical clobetasol on oral mucosa: topical clobetasol systemic absorption. J Oral Pathol Med 2012;41:255–60.
43. Conrotto D, Carrozzo M, Ubertalli AV, et al. Dramatic increase of tacrolimus plasma concentration during topical treatment for oral graft-versus-host disease. Transplantation 2006;82:1113–5.
44. Bijl P, van Eyk A. Human vaginal mucosa as a model of buccal mucosa for in vitro permeability studies: an overview. Curr Drug Deliv 2004;1:129–35.
45. Schimmer AD, Quatermain M, Imrie K, et al. Ovarian function after autologous bone marrow transplantation. J Clin Oncol 1998;16:2359–63.
46. Hamilton BK, Goje O, Savani BN, et al. Clinical management of genital chronic GvHD. Bone Marrow Transplant 2017. http://dx.doi.org/10.1038/bmt.2016.315.
47. Pandit L, Ouslander JG. Postmenopausal vaginal atrophy and atrophic vaginitis. Am J Med Sci 1997;314:228–31.
48. Muhleisen AL, Herbst-Kralovetz MM. Menopause and the vaginal microbiome. Maturitas 2016;91:42–50.
49. Shen J, Song N, Williams CJ, et al. Effects of low dose estrogen therapy on the vaginal microbiomes of women with atrophic vaginitis. Sci Rep 2016;6:24380.
50. Notelovitz M. Urogenital aging: solutions in clinical practice. Int J Gynaecol Obstet 1997;59:S35–9.
51. Management of symptomatic vulvovaginal atrophy: 2013 position statement of The North American Menopause Society. Menopause 2013;20:888–902.
52. Briedite I, Ancane G, Ancans A, et al. Insufficient assessment of sexual dysfunction: a problem in gynecological practice. Medicina (Kaunas) 2013;49:315–20.
53. Schlosser BJ. Missing genital lichen sclerosus in patients with morphea: Don't ask? Don't tell? Arch Dermatol 2012;148:28.
54. Bhatia S, Louie AD, Bhatia R, et al. Solid cancers after bone marrow transplantation. J Clin Oncol 2001;19:464–71.
55. Savani BN, Stratton P, Shenoy A, et al. Increased risk of cervical dysplasia in long-term survivors of allogeneic stem cell transplantation—implications for screening and HPV vaccination. Biol Blood Marrow Transplant 2008;14:1072–5.
56. Grulich AE, van Leeuwen MT, Falster MO, et al. Incidence of cancers in people with HIV/AIDS compared with immunosuppressed transplant recipients: a meta-analysis. Lancet 2007;370:59–67.

57. Sri T, Merideth MA, Pulanic TK, et al. Human papillomavirus reactivation following treatment of genital graft-versus-host disease. Transpl Infect Dis 2013;15: E148–51.
58. Savani BN, Griffith ML, Jagasia S, et al. How I treat late effects in adults after allogeneic stem cell transplantation. Blood 2011;117:3002–9.

Vulvodynia
Diagnosis and Management

Amy L. Stenson, MD, MSc

KEYWORDS

- Vulvodynia • Vulvar pain • Sexual pain • Vestibulodynia

KEY POINTS

- Vulvodynia is defined as vulvar pain that has been present for at least 3 months, with no clear identifiable cause. Classification of vulvodynia is based on 4 factors: site of pain (generalized, localized, or mixed); whether it is provoked, spontaneous, or mixed; onset (primary vs secondary); and temporal pattern.
- History and physical examination should include a thorough medical history with specific focus on pain history, sexual history, and psychosocial evaluation; careful visual inspection of the vulva; cotton swab testing, to identify the location of pain; a sensitive speculum examination, to evaluate for discharge or any abnormalities of the vaginal mucosa; and a musculoskeletal examination with a focus on evaluation of the pelvic floor muscles. It is important to rule out other conditions that may be contributing to pain before making the diagnosis of vulvodynia.
- Treatment of vulvodynia is optimized with a multidisciplinary approach that includes psychotherapy, pelvic physical therapy, and medical therapy. Treatment of any type of vulvodynia should be individualized.
- There is a lack of high-quality data to support medical treatment options for vulvodynia. The following medications can be considered based on expert opinion and limited data until better evidence is available:
  - Generalized vulvodynia: oral neuromodulators (eg, tricyclic antidepressants [TCAs], serotonin or norepinephrine reuptake inhibitors, gabapentin, and pregabalin).
  - Provoked vestibulodynia (PVD): compounded topical therapies (eg, Lidocaine, TCAs, baclofen, gabapentin, and capsaicin) and surgery.
- Vestibulectomy (surgical excision) performed by an experienced provider can be very effective treatment of PVD. This may be an excellent option for patients who have not responded to other treatment options.

No disclosures.
Program in Vulvar Health, Department of Obstetrics and Gynecology, Oregon Health & Science University, 3181 Southwest Sam Jackson Park Road, Mail Code: UHN-50, Portland, OR 97239, USA
E-mail address: stenson@ohsu.edu

Obstet Gynecol Clin N Am 44 (2017) 493–508
http://dx.doi.org/10.1016/j.ogc.2017.05.008
0889-8545/17/© 2017 Elsevier Inc. All rights reserved.
obgyn.theclinics.com

INTRODUCTION

Vulvar pain is a common gynecologic complaint. Studies of the general population have estimated that chronic vulvar pain is present in 8% to 15%[1-3] of reproductive aged women and that this health issue may cost society somewhere between 31 to 72 billion dollars annually in the United States.[4] Many women with chronic vulvar pain report a poor quality of life, seek multiple health care providers, are frequently misdiagnosed, and use multiple treatment modalities before experiencing any degree of symptom relief. It is, therefore, important for any women's health practitioner to appreciate this condition and have a basic understanding of the diagnosis and management options.

The International Society for the Study of Vulvar Disease (ISSVD) along with the International Society for the Study of Women's Sexual Health, and the International Pelvic Pain Society adopted a new classification system for vulvar pain in 2015.[5] This system acknowledges the complexity of making these diagnoses and broadly divides the vulvar pain conditions into 2 main groups: vulvar pain caused by a specific disorder (**Table 1**) and vulvodynia. Vulvodynia is defined as vulvar pain that has been present for at least 3 months, with no clear identifiable cause. It is described by the following key characteristics:

- Location: localized (eg, vestibule, clitoris), generalized, or mixed
- Provocation: spontaneous, provoked (eg, touch, insertional), or mixed
- Onset: primary (symptoms have always been present) or secondary (symptoms developed later after a period of normal functioning)
- Temporal pattern: intermittent, persistent, constant, immediate, or delayed.

The new classification includes a list of potentially associated factors (eg, psychosocial factors, musculoskeletal issues, comorbidities, genetics, inflammation, neuroproliferation), suggesting that vulvodynia is likely not a single disease but represents the overlap of several disease processes. The characterization of vulvar pain using this criteria allows for the appreciation of several common specific subtypes of vulvodynia. This article focuses on the diagnosis and management of the 2 most common subtypes of vulvodynia:

1. Provoked vestibulodynia (PVD), defined as localized, provoked vulvodynia of the (vulvar) vestibule
2. Generalized vulvodynia (GD), defined as unprovoked vulvodynia of the entire vulva.

Table 1	
Examples of vulvar pain caused by a specific disorder	
Category	**Examples**
Infectious	Recurrent candidiasis, herpes simplex virus
Inflammatory	Lichen planus, lichen sclerosus
Neoplastic	Paget disease, squamous cell carcinoma
Neurologic	Nerve compression, neuroma, postherpetic neuralgia
Trauma	Obstetric injury, female genital cutting
Iatrogenic	Radiation, postoperative
Hormonal	Genitourinary syndrome of menopause, lactational amenorrhea

Modified from Bornstein J, Goldstein AT, Stockdale CK, et al. 2015 ISSVD, ISSWSH and IPPS consensus terminology and classification of persistent vulvar pain and vulvodynia. Obstet Gynecol 2016;127(4):747; with permission.

CAUSE OF VULVODYNIA

The cause of vulvodynia is not well understood; however, most experts agree that it is most likely multifactorial and differs by subtype.[6,7] Epidemiologic studies suggest a link between a history of vulvovaginal infection, particularly recurrent or severe infections, and the subsequent development of vulvodynia. Histologic studies in women with PVD compared with controls have demonstrated neuroproliferation of the vestibule, increased lymphocytes and mast cells, and increased proinflammatory cytokines,[6,8–12] though results have not been consistent across all studies. GD is considered a centrally mediated pain condition similar to other chronic pain conditions (eg, fibromyalgia) by many experts and there have not been any histologic studies to date. Some have suggested hormonal alteration (oral contraceptive pill use, menopause) as part of the etiologic pathway in vulvodynia.[7] Genetic predisposition is suggested by the observation that PVD clusters in families.[13] There is consensus that further study is critical to better understanding the pathophysiology and cause of vulvodynia.

DIAGNOSIS
History

The diagnosis of vulvodynia is primarily based on clinical history coupled with physical examination and is largely a diagnosis of exclusion. It is important to identify and treat specific disorders that may be contributing to pain before making a diagnosis of vulvodynia. A thorough evaluation of the patient's pain history, sexual history, psychosocial situation, medical history, and physical examination are key aspects to correctly diagnosing and managing vulvodynia. Recently, a tool called the Vulvar Pain Assessment Questionnaire (VPAQ) was developed as a disease-specific set of measurement scales designed to capture the biopsychosocial nature of vulvodynia. Specifically, the VPAQ assesses pain quality, the temporal nature of the pain, associated symptoms, pain intensity, emotional or cognitive functioning, physical functioning, coping strategies, and interpersonal functioning.[14] Additionally, the ISSVD has developed a questionnaire that patients can fill out before their appointments to enable this process (available online at http://women4real.com/wp-content/uploads/2013/09/Vulvodynia-Clinical-questionnaire.pdf).

Establishing a trusting relationship is of paramount importance, particularly because many women have suffered with their condition for long periods of time, seen multiple providers in the past, and have unsuccessfully tried different treatment strategies. It is important to address the women's feelings and allow for adequate time to gain a complete picture of the patient's problem. Assuring confidentiality and privacy, supporting any emotions that come up, allowing time for the patient to tell her whole story, and communicating clearly with empathy are some practices that can help build a professional and empathetic relationship with the patient. In settings in which time is limited, it may be useful to reassure the patient of the importance of the problem and then schedule her for additional follow-up at a time when a more comprehensive assessment can be completed. Understanding what the patient views as her primary problem and what her expectations are around management can help to facilitate patient-centered care that best aligns with her goals. For example, a woman may report generalized burning pain, low libido, and dyspareunia and be most worried about her relationship with her husband, in which case focusing initially on relationship counseling while working through the other issues may be the most important aspect of treatment to her.

Pain History

Characterizing the patient's pain by performing a detailed pain history is crucial to the diagnosis of vulvodynia. The interview should elicit location, quality, intensity, and duration of pain episodes. Additional questions that may be helpful include

- How long has she had pain?
- Has she always had pain or did it start after a period of no pain (primary vs secondary)?
- What other conditions or clinical symptoms accompanied the onset of pain (eg, yeast infection, initiation of a new medication)?
- Are there things that provoke or alleviate the pain?
- How much impact does the pain have on daily life?

Women with PVD will frequently report pain at the opening to the vagina with vaginal penetration (eg, tampon use, intercourse), whereas women with GD will often report constant soreness, burning, or irritating pain throughout the entire vulva.

Sexual History

A sensitive and thorough sexual history reassures the patient that her physician understands the complexity of the problem and will work to address all facets of her issue. It may be useful to start with evaluation of her current sexuality, including desire, arousal, orgasm, sexual frequency, sexual practices (ie, use of sex toys or vibrators; anal, vaginal, or oral sex; use of lubrication), and sexual satisfaction. Understanding the patient's relationships and level of intimacy can provide insight into how they are coping and the level of support that they have from their partner. Patients experiencing relationship issues may have difficulty discussing sexuality and may benefit from discussion of related issues such as avoidance behaviors, conflict, or negative partner responses. Patients who have a history of sexual abuse or negative sexual experiences, particularly any childhood trauma, may need additional time to discuss this history and will likely benefit from a follow-up visit or referral for further management. Many women with vulvodynia will feel distress around issues of sexuality and may have significant psychological impact as a result. Anxiety, depression, hypervigilance, fear of pain, and catastrophizing are examples of common psychological issues that women with vulvodynia may face, and addressing these can help women in the healing process.

Medical History

The medical history should be comprehensive and pay particular attention to the following:

- Comorbid conditions (eg, fibromyalgia, temporomandibular joint, and other chronic pain conditions)
- Mental health issues (eg, anxiety, depression)
- Medication use (eg, hormonal therapy, topical genital therapy)
- Associated symptoms (eg, bowel and bladder dysfunction)
- Infection history (eg, frequent urinary tract infections, recurrent yeast)
- Musculoskeletal history (eg, previous surgery or injury affecting the pelvis, hip, or sacrum)
- Exercise or activity level (eg, inability to ride a bike due to pain)
- Social support system.

Research shows that women with vulvodynia have higher rates of comorbid pain conditions and show substantial alterations in pain pathways peripherally and centrally.[15,16] Many patients with vulvodynia have suffered with their condition for many years and previous treatment attempts and outcomes should be documented. Patients also frequently seek complementary and alternative methods for treating pain, such as acupuncture or herbal remedies, but may leave them out of the history unless this is asked directly.

Physical Examination

A focused physical and thorough pelvic examination is critical to the diagnosis of vulvodynia. It is important to understand and acknowledge that patients may have high anxiety around genital touch due to a history of dyspareunia or painful past examinations. Involving patients in their own examination using techniques such as the interactive educational pelvic examination may be helpful.[17] This technique involves educating the patient about her anatomy, explaining each step of the examination to the patient, encouraging the patient to observe the examination with a hand-held mirror, and allowing time for questions and information exchange.

Vulvar Inspection

The vulvar skin and vaginal mucosa should be carefully inspected to evaluate for abnormalities such as hypopigmentation, fissuring, scarring, ulceration, or neoplasia. Some practitioners advocate routine use of colposcopy of the vulva or vulvoscopy for patients with vulvodynia because it may enhance identification of subtle findings (eg, inflammation, fissures, and lichenification); however, application of acetic acid increases discomfort and is not necessary. If abnormalities are present, a biopsy may be considered for tissue diagnosis to rule out conditions such as lichen sclerosus, lichen planus, low-grade or high-grade squamous intraepithelial lesions, differentiated vulvar intraepithelial neoplasia, or squamous cell cancer. This is typically done using a 3 to 4 mm punch biopsy, a snip biopsy, or an excisional biopsy. There is very little utility in a biopsy of normal appearing skin and this should be avoided. Erythema of the vulva or vestibule may be present in vulvodynia but is not part of the diagnostic criteria. Bright erythema of the vestibule, particularly in the area of the Bartholin duct openings is very commonly seen in PVD and does not warrant a biopsy.

Sensory Examination: Cotton Swab Test

The next step of the examination involves systematic palpation of all areas of the anogenital region, most commonly by using a moistened cotton swab to apply light touch to each area (ie, the cotton swab test[18]). The examination starts with areas less likely to be painful, specifically the medial thighs, buttocks, and mons pubis, allowing the patient to adjust to the examination. It then proceeds with palpation of the labia majora, perineum, clitoris, and the labia minora lateral to Hart's line (**Fig. 1**). Areas that are not midline should be palpated bilaterally. Pain with palpation of these areas suggests a more generalized process, and care should be taken to evaluate closely for infection, dermatoses, or other causes. The next step involves palpation of the vestibule, which is the mucosa that lies between Hart's line and the hymen. There is variation in how this test is performed. The most common approach involves light palpation with the cotton swab at 5 to 6 points on the vestibule: at the ostia of the Skene glands lateral to the urethra, between the urethra and clitoris at 12 o'clock, at the ostia of the Bartholin glands at 4 and 8 o'clock, and at the fossa navicularis at 6 o'clock. Patients are asked to report pain intensity using a numerical rating scale (NRS) of 0 to 10 or by simply reporting yes or no if they are experiencing pain.

In my practice I perform the cotton swab test on the vestibule at 6 points and ask patients to report pain using the NRS. I then apply 4% liquid lidocaine with 2 soaked,

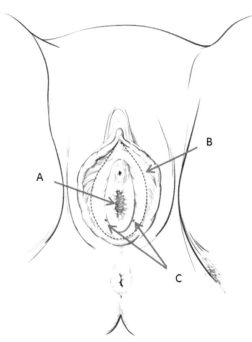

Fig. 1. The vulva. The vestibule is the region between (A) the hymen and (B) Hart's line (*dotted line*). (C) The opening of the Bartholin ducts can be seen bilaterally at 4 and 8 o'clock. (*Courtesy of* Robin Jensen, Portland, OR.)

large cotton swabs for 3 minutes and re-evaluate the extent to which this changes the patient's pain rating (**Fig. 2**). This last step, re-evaluating after the application of 4% liquid lidocaine, is not included in the classic description of the cotton swab test but has been described.[19] Patients with PVD will report pain with touch to the vestibule

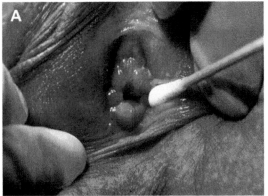
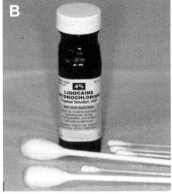

Fig. 2. (*A*) The cotton swab test being performed at 4 o'clock on the vulvar vestibule. The test is performed using a gentle rolling motion at each point on the vestibule (12, 2, 4, 6, 8, and 10 o'clock). Pain is reported using a numeric rating scale 0 to 10. When significant vestibular pain is reported, (*B*) 4% topical lidocaine solution is applied for 3 minutes and the test repeated (ie, the lidocaine test).

and normal sensation lateral to Hart's line. In my experience, they will also typically report a 50% to 90% decrease in pain scores on the NRS after application of lidocaine. Patients with GD are unlikely to have additional pain elicited by the examination but may report that the areas being palpated are where they experience pain.

Speculum Examination

Following the cotton swab test, the vagina should be evaluated using a speculum with sensitivity to the pain that inserting the speculum may cause the patient. Many practitioners will use a pediatric Graves or small Pederson speculum and minimize contact with the vestibule by inserting the speculum through the hymenal ring. In my practice the speculum examination is performed after application of 4% liquid lidocaine to the painful vestibule and this results in a more comfortable and useful speculum examination. This practice also helps me distinguish vestibular pain from vaginal or musculoskeletal pain. Once the speculum is inserted, the vaginal mucosa should be carefully inspected for atrophy, erythema, ulcerations, erosions, abnormal discharge, and architectural changes or scarring. Any discharge can be collected for evaluation (see later discussion).

Manual Examination

Manual examination of the pelvic floor muscles, bladder trigone, urethra, and the pudendal nerve as it enters Alcock canal can be performed using 1 finger instead of 2, with attention to avoiding touch to the vestibule to minimize discomfort. When using lidocaine as previously described, this is often not necessary unless there is significant contracture of the vaginal muscles. A bimanual examination may be performed to evaluate the uterus and adnexa if there is concern for disease such as pelvic inflammatory disease or endometriosis. Evaluation of the pelvic floor, trunk and lower extremity musculature and treatment of pelvic floor dysfunction is described in detail (see Stephanie A. Prendergast's article, "Pelvic Floor Physical Therapy for Vulvodynia: A Clinician's Guide," in this issue). Most patients with vulvodynia, particularly PVD, have increased pelvic floor muscle tone and poor muscle control, thus addressing this aspect of the disease is critical to the ultimate success of treatment.

Laboratory and Point-of-Care Testing

Performing a wet mount, potassium hydroxide (KOH) prep, and vaginal pH can be helpful to exclude infectious causes, such as candidiasis, trichomoniasis, and bacterial vaginosis (BV); or inflammatory conditions, such as lichen planus and desquamative inflammatory vaginitis (DIV). Although rapid point-of-care tests can identify common infectious causes, a wet mount can provide additional information (eg, presence of increased white blood cells and parabasal cells in DIV). It may also be helpful to send cultures for fungal speciation and sensitivity if there is a suspicion for refractory or recurrent yeast. Normal vaginal pH is 3.5 to 4.5; elevations in pH greater than 4.7 are suggestive of BV, trichomoniasis, or an inflammatory condition. An elevation is also noted in hypoestrogenic states. Patients with vulvodynia (PVD or GD) will most likely have a normal pH and wet mount. If vulvodynia is suspected and a patient is diagnosed with candidiasis or BV, the infection should be treated and the patient re-evaluated in 6 to 8 weeks to allow for the inflammation to normalize. Keep in mind that BV is not a painful condition but may add to a confusing clinical picture and, therefore, it is best to treat BV before definitively diagnosing vulvodynia. In general, bacterial culture of the vagina is not helpful and is not recommended.

See **Fig. 3** for a synopsis of the key features of the history and physical examination that differentiate GV from PVD.

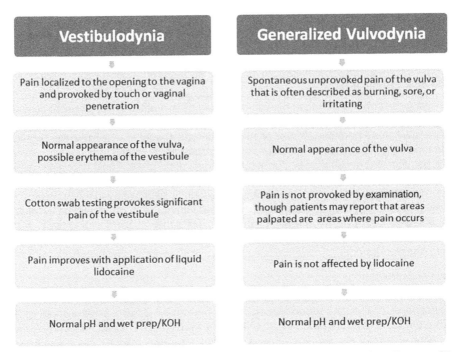

Fig. 3. Comparison of key aspects of the history and physical examination in PVD versus GD. KOH, potassium hydroxide.

Management

Optimal management of vulvodynia varies by subtype but, in general, requires a multidisciplinary approach that includes promotion of vulvar health, psychological treatment, physical therapy, and medical therapy. Data are limited on the efficacy of many of the most common therapies and treatment decisions are, therefore, guided by clinical experience or expert opinion, and tailored to individual patients.[20] A recent study demonstrated spontaneous resolution of pain in 22% of patients untreated over 2 years. Remission was more common in women who did not have pain with intercourse and in those who reported less severe pain initially.[21] It may be useful to discuss these factors from the onset to help patients understand that improvement can be a slow process, and finding the right treatment may require trialing several different therapies. Before starting any new treatments, it may be wise to have the patient stop all topical vulvar therapies because they may be contributing to vulvar irritant dermatitis. Some practitioners start with less invasive treatments (eg, counseling, physical therapy) and move toward more invasive treatment (eg, medications, surgery), depending on response. Many consider concurrent multidisciplinary therapy the best approach because the woman affected by vulvodynia often is suffering physically, emotionally, relationally, and sexually. A multidisciplinary approach is a holistic approach that considers all the different ways that vulvodynia has affected her life (**Fig. 4**).

Promotion of Vulvar Health

Contact with some products can cause irritation and pain of the vulva. These may include soaps, creams, fragrances, tight-fitting clothing, douches, deodorants,

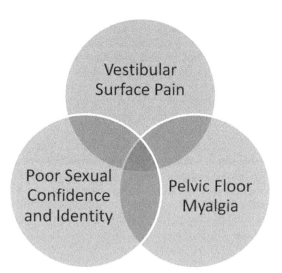

Fig. 4. It is important to recognize and address the interaction of vestibular surface pain, pelvic floor myalgia, and the development of poor sexual confidence or identity in patients with vestibulodynia. Failure to address any component will frequently result in suboptimal treatment.

synthetic lubricants, tampons, pads, and commercial vaginal wipes. Avoidance of these irritants is supported by the American College of Obstetricians and Gynecologists and can lead to improved symptoms for some patients. In addition, patients can be encouraged to wash the vulva with water alone, wear loose fitting cotton undergarments during the day and none while asleep, use a nonirritating lubricant for intercourse (eg, coconut oil if not using condoms for contraception), avoid use of hair dryers, pat the area dry after bathing, and switch to all-cotton menstrual pads. Self-care practices that may provide symptomatic relief include applying cool compresses to the vulva for 10 to 15 minutes or soaking in an Epsom salt or colloidal oatmeal bath. Good vulvar hygiene and self-care is a reasonable first step that patients can implement immediately and may lead to improvement of symptoms.[22]

Psychological Interventions

The goals of psychotherapy include decreasing pain, strengthening romantic relationships, and restoring sexual function by focusing on the thoughts, emotions, behaviors, and ways that couples interact in the setting of genital pain. Counseling may take an individual, couple, or group format, and there are advantages with each. The most commonly used form of psychotherapy is cognitive-behavioral therapy (CBT). Group-based CBT has been evaluated in several clinical trials, shown to significantly decrease pain during intercourse at 6-month follow-up, and this effect was sustained over long-term follow-up at 2.5 years.[23,24] Women who participated in therapy reported high satisfaction, less pain catastrophizing, and better sexual function. Psychotherapy (individualized, couple, and group therapy) is a validated, safe, noninvasive option for treatment of vulvodynia and should be highly considered as a critical aspect of treatment.[20,25] Insurance coverage may be an issue for some patients; however, many insurance groups do provide this benefit and women should be encouraged to participate if able.

Alternative Therapy

The use of alternative therapy among patients is widespread, but there are few data to support efficacy.[20] There are uncontrolled pilot studies suggesting improvement in pain with acupuncture and hypnosis and a small wait-list controlled study of acupuncture that showed improvement in vulvar pain, dyspareunia, and overall sexual function.[26] The risks of adverse effects are minimal and patients may prefer to try these techniques before embarking on surgical or medical management.

Physical Therapy

Pelvic floor physical therapy is a cornerstone of treatment of women with vulvodynia because most women have concomitant pelvic floor muscle dysfunction (vaginismus) as a compensatory mechanism to avoid pain (see Stephanie A. Prendergast's article, "Pelvic Floor Physical Therapy for Vulvodynia: A Clinician's Guide," in this issue). Failure to address pelvic floor dysfunction in patients with vulvodynia is likely to result in suboptimal treatment.

MEDICAL MANAGEMENT OF VULVODYNIA
Local Therapy

The 3 main local therapy types that have been used for PVD are antinociceptive agents (anesthetics such as lidocaine, capsaicin, and botulinum), anti-inflammatory agents (corticosteroids, interferon, cromolyn, and lysate), and compounded neuromodulators or combinations (tricyclic antidepressants [TCAs], gabapentin, and baclofen) (**Table 2**). Although many case series have suggested promising results, clinical trials of topical agents to date have shown limited or no long-term efficacy and these agents are not recommended for curative treatment of PVD.[20,25,27,28] Similarly, injection of botulinum toxin A, corticosteroids, and interferon have very limited data to support use and are not recommended. Recently, hormonal topical therapy (0.01% estradiol and 0.1% testosterone) was reported to significantly decrease pain for women with PVD who were on oral contraceptive pills when their pain started, but this was a

Table 2
Commonly used topical medications for the management of provoked vestibulodynia

Name	Dosing	Efficacy
Lidocaine 5% (cream or ointment)	Applied daily	No clear benefit vs placebo in 2 RCTs; both groups improved[27,28] Descriptive study showed improved pain and frequency of sex
Gabapentin 2%–6% (cream)	Applied daily	No RCTs Descriptive study showed improvement in pain and increased frequency of intercourse
Amitriptyline 2% or baclofen 2% (cream)	Applied daily	No RCTs Descriptive study reported improved pain
Estrogen 0.01% and/or testosterone 0.05% (cream)	Applied daily	No RCTs Case series demonstrated significant decrease in pain[29]
Capsaicin 0.025%–0.05% (cream)	Applied daily for 20 min and then removed	No RCTs. Observational studies demonstrated decreased pain

case series and further data are needed from RCTs before this can be strongly recommended.[29]

Use of a topical anesthetic such as lidocaine can provide the patient with temporary relief of pain. This can be demonstrated in the office by applying lidocaine to the vestibule and having the patient report pain with touch before and after using the lidocaine. For patients with PVD, care must be taken to ensure that the lidocaine is applied to all of the areas that are painful and it sometimes tricky to ensure that the lidocaine penetrates the crevice between the hymen and vestibule, particularly at the opening to the Bartholin duct. The author's practice offers lidocaine to patients to use as needed and many patients will apply this before or after intercourse, when exercising, or anytime that they experience increased pain. Preferred formulations are a 4% viscous lidocaine solution, a 5% lidocaine ointment, and a 2% lidocaine gel. There are many different formulations of lidocaine. Insurance coverage, availability, and cost may necessitate trialing several to find the formulation that is well-tolerated and affordable for the patient. Topical lidocaine application is very safe, though there are reports of toxicity in patients who have applied copious amounts of topical lidocaine to a large surface area of the body. Care should be taken to use the appropriate amount to cover only the painful region (vestibule). Maximum recommended amount is 4.5 mg/kg every 3 hours, which is much higher than the amount needed to cover the vestibule.

When using a topical therapy it is important to consider the vehicle for medication application because many creams contain preservatives and stabilizer that can produce burning. An ointment or liquid may be better tolerated, or a compounding pharmacy can work with practitioners to find a media that is appropriate and least likely to be irritating. It is often useful to call the compounding pharmacist to discuss options.

Oral Medication

There are several oral medications that can be used in the treatment of vulvodynia. Use of these agents in vulvodynia is based on their successful use in other chronic neuropathic pain states (eg, fibromyalgia). These include TCAs (eg, amitriptyline, nortriptyline, and desipramine), serotonin or norepinephrine reuptake inhibitors (SNRIs; eg, duloxetine), and anticonvulsants (eg, gabapentin, pregabalin) (**Table 3**). Treatment with any of these agents requires attention to side effects and potential drug interactions. In general, doses should be started low and titrated up gradually to allow tolerance to the side effects.

Table 3		
Commonly used oral medications for management of generalized vulvodynia		
Name	**Dosing**	**Titration**

TCAs
    Amitriptyline
    Nortriptyline
    Desipramine
	10–100 mg/d (average 50–75 mg/d)	Start at 10–25 mg and titrate up by 10–25 mg every 7 d to max dose

Duloxetine	20–60 mg/d	Start at 20 mg and titrate up by 20 mg/d every 7 d to max dose
Gabapentin	100–3600 mg/d in 3 divided doses	Start at 100 mg and titrate up by 100 mg/d every 5–7 d if well-tolerated
Pregabalin	150–300 mg/d in 2–3 divided doses	Start at 150 mg and titrate up by to 300 mg after 1 wk if well-tolerated

A review of the literature regarding use of TCAs for treatment of vulvodynia in 2013 evaluated the existing studies to date, which included only 2 randomized clinical trials (RCTs) and a total of 13 reports or studies. They concluded that there is a paucity of high-quality data in this arena. One RCT indicated that oral TCA therapy is no better than placebo in treating PVD[28] and, therefore, it was recommended that oral antidepressant therapy not be used for treatment of PVD.[30] There were too few data to draw conclusions for GV.[30]

A similar review of anticonvulsants was conducted in 2013 and, although most of the included studies demonstrated a 50% to 80% satisfaction with pain improvement, the studies were of poor methodological quality, not placebo controlled, not stratified by vulvodynia subtype, and the analysis concluded that there was insufficient evidence to recommend any of the anticonvulsants for vulvodynia management.[31] That report advocates using these agents for refractory cases based on the clinical expertise of the gynecologist as part of patient-centered comprehensive care. Some investigators recommend awaiting the results of a multicenter RCT before prescribing these medications.

In my practice, I typically do not recommend any oral medications for PVD unless the patient has comorbid conditions that would benefit from treatment. However, I find oral medications useful for patients with GV. I will start with a low dose and titrate up to the lowest dose that has been shown to be effective for management of chronic pain, have the patient stay at that dose for at least 2 weeks, and then titrate up over several weeks to the maximal dose (see **Table 3**).

Surgical Management of Provoked Vestibulodynia

Surgical management is currently the most effective therapy to treat PVD with success rates of 60% to 100% reported.[32] Evidence is limited to case series and prospective cohorts. To date, there have been no RCTs, studies vary in how they measure outcomes, and there are variable follow-up times. Vulvar vestibulectomy was first described in 1981 by Woodruff and colleagues.[33] The steps of their procedure include excision of a semicircular segment of the perineal skin, the posterior vulvar vestibule, and the posterior hymenal ring. The vaginal mucosa is undermined for 3 cm and approximated to the perineum.

There are several variations of the procedure. A complete vestibulectomy involves removal of all of the vestibular mucosa, including the portion adjacent to the urethra. Modifications of the procedure include limiting excision to the posterior vestibule or mapping the excision to excise only the mucosa that is painful on examination.[34]

The author's practice recommends surgery primarily for patients with provoked localized pain of the vestibule that resolves or significantly improves with application of lidocaine to the vestibule. Lidocaine penetrates the superficial layers of the mucosa. The author believes that resolution of pain with lidocaine application suggests that surgical removal of that tissue is more likely to successfully treat these patients. The author's practice adheres to a modified vestibulectomy technique based on pain mapping that has been verified at multiple visits (at a minimum, the initial visit and just before surgery) (**Fig. 5**). The author has observed that surgical outcomes are better when coupled with psychotherapy and pelvic physical therapy, and recommends them before and after surgery in most cases.[35]

Surgical management is not effective for GD but could be considered for patients with mixed vulvodynia, provided that the patient is well counseled and understands what component of her pain is likely to be addressed by surgery, and that the surgeon is experienced with pain mapping and performing the appropriate surgical procedure.

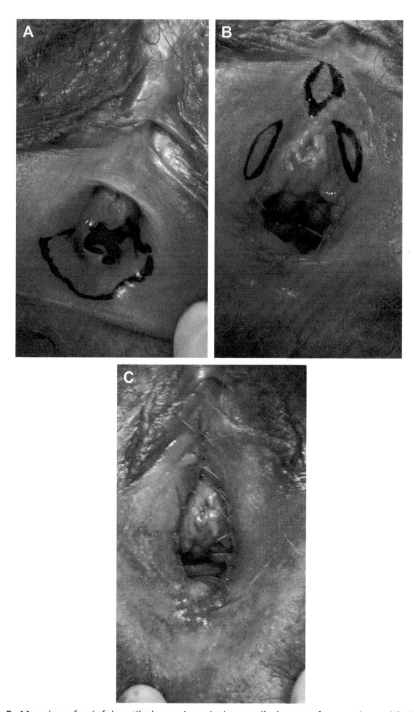

Fig. 5. Mapping of painful vestibular regions during vestibulectomy for a patient with PVD. (*A*) The region of pain in the posterior vestibule between Hart's line and the hymenal ridge. (*B*) Islands of tissue for excision in the anterior vestibule that the patient reports as most painful. (*C*) The final surgical result.

Summary of Treatment Options

The following are recommended as options for treatment of vulvodynia, acknowledging the lack of high-quality data to support these recommendations:

- A multidisciplinary, individualized, and patient-centered approach
- Practices that promote vulvar health
- Psychotherapy (individualized, group, and/or couple therapy)
- Pelvic physical therapy (see Stephanie A. Prendergast's article, "Pelvic Floor Physical Therapy for Vulvodynia: A Clinician's Guide," in this issue).
- Topical lidocaine to reduce pain as needed, particularly for PVD
- Oral neuromodulators (TCAs, SNRIs, or gabapentin) for GV
- Surgical management (vestibulectomy) for PVD
- Alternative therapy has little risk (acupuncture, hypnosis) and can be considered.

SUMMARY

Vulvodynia is an important women's health issue that significantly affects sexual function and quality of life. Women will benefit from a multidimensional approach to therapy and it may be useful to help set realistic expectations about treatment time course and outcome. More data are urgently needed around management options for vulvodynia.

REFERENCES

1. Reed BD, Harlow SD, Sen A, et al. Prevalence and demographic characteristics of vulvodynia in a population-based sample. Am J Obstet Gynecol 2012;206(2):170.e1-9.
2. Harlow BL, Stewart EG. A population-based assessment of chronic unexplained vulvar pain: have we underestimated the prevalence of vulvodynia? J Am Med Womens Assoc 2003;58(2):82–8.
3. Arnold LD, Bachmann GA, Rosen R, et al. Assessment of vulvodynia symptoms in a sample of US women: a prevalence survey with a nested case control study. Am J Obstet Gynecol 2007;196(2):128.e1-6.
4. Xie Y, Shi L, Xiong X, et al. Economic burden and quality of life of vulvodynia in the United States. Curr Med Res Opin 2012;28(4):601–8.
5. Bornstein J, Goldstein AT, Stockdale CK, et al. 2015 ISSVD, ISSWSH and IPPS consensus terminology and classification of persistent vulvar pain and vulvodynia. Obstet Gynecol 2016;127(4):745–51.
6. Havemann LM, Cool DR, Gagneux P, et al. Vulvodynia: what we know and where we should be going. J Low Genit Tract Dis 2017;21(2):150–6.
7. Pukall CF, Goldstein AT, Bergeron S, et al. Vulvodynia: definition, prevalence, impact, and pathophysiological factors. J Sex Med 2016;13(3):291–304.
8. Leclair CM, Leeborg NJ, Jacobson-Dunlop E, et al. CD4-positive T-cell recruitment in primary-provoked localized vulvodynia: potential insights into disease triggers. J Low Genit Tract Dis 2014;18(2):195–201.
9. Goetsch MF, Morgan TK, Korcheva VB, et al. Histologic and receptor analysis of primary and secondary vestibulodynia and controls: a prospective study. Am J Obstet Gynecol 2010;202(6):614.e1-8.
10. Leclair CM, Goetsch MF, Korcheva VB, et al. Differences in primary compared with secondary vestibulodynia by immunohistochemistry. Obstet Gynecol 2011;117(6):1307–13.

11. Leclair CM, Goetsch MF, Li H, et al. Histopathologic characteristics of menopausal vestibulodynia. Obstet Gynecol 2013;122(4):787–93.

12. Falsetta ML, Foster DC, Bonham AD, et al. A review of the available clinical therapies for vulvodynia management and new data implicating proinflammatory mediators in pain elicitation. BJOG 2017;124(2):210–8.

13. Morgan TK, Allen-Brady KL, Monson MA, et al. Familiality analysis of provoked vestibulodynia treated by vestibulectomy supports genetic predisposition. Am J Obstet Gynecol 2016;214(5):609.e1-7.

14. Dargie E, Holden RR, Pukall CF. The Vulvar Pain Assessment Questionnaire inventory. Pain 2016;157(12):2672–86.

15. Gupta A, Rapkin AJ, Gill Z, et al. Disease-related differences in resting-state networks: a comparison between localized provoked vulvodynia, irritable bowel syndrome, and healthy control subjects. Pain 2015;156(5):809–19.

16. Reed BD, Legocki LJ, Plegue MA, et al. Factors associated with vulvodynia incidence. Obstet Gynecol 2014;123(2 Pt 1):225–31.

17. Huber JD, Pukall CF, Boyer SC, et al. "Just relax": physicians' experiences with women who are difficult or impossible to examine gynecologically. J Sex Med 2009;6(3):791–9.

18. Friedrich EG Jr. Vulvar vestibulitis syndrome. J Reprod Med 1987;32(2):110–4.

19. Goetsch MF, Lim JY, Caughey AB. A practical solution for dyspareunia in breast cancer survivors: a randomized controlled trial. J Clin Oncol 2015;33(30): 3394–400.

20. Goldstein AT, Pukall CF, Brown C, et al. Vulvodynia: assessment and treatment. J Sex Med 2016;13(4):572–90.

21. Reed BD, Haefner HK, Sen A, et al. Vulvodynia incidence and remission rates among adult women: a 2-year follow-up study. Obstet Gynecol 2008;112(2 Pt 1):231–7.

22. Committee opinion no 673 summary: persistent vulvar pain. Obstet Gynecol 2016;128(3):676–7.

23. Bergeron S, Khalife S, Glazer HI, et al. Surgical and behavioral treatments for vestibulodynia: two-and-one-half year follow-up and predictors of outcome. Obstet Gynecol 2008;111(1):159–66.

24. Bergeron S, Khalife S, Dupuis MJ, et al. A randomized clinical trial comparing group cognitive-behavioral therapy and a topical steroid for women with dyspareunia. J Consult Clin Psychol 2016;84(3):259–68.

25. Stockdale CK, Lawson HW. 2013 vulvodynia guideline update. J Low Genit Tract Dis 2014;18(2):93–100.

26. Schlaeger JM, Xu N, Mejta CL, et al. Acupuncture for the treatment of vulvodynia: a randomized wait-list controlled pilot study. J Sex Med 2015;12(4):1019–27.

27. Danielsson I, Torstensson T, Brodda-Jansen G, et al. EMG biofeedback versus topical lidocaine gel: a randomized study for the treatment of women with vulvar vestibulitis. Acta Obstet Gynecol Scand 2006;85(11):1360–7.

28. Foster DC, Kotok MB, Huang LS, et al. Oral desipramine and topical lidocaine for vulvodynia: a randomized controlled trial. Obstet Gynecol 2010;116(3):583–93.

29. Burrows LJ, Goldstein AT. The treatment of vestibulodynia with topical estradiol and testosterone. Sex Med 2013;1(1):30–3.

30. Leo RJ, Dewani S. A systematic review of the utility of antidepressant pharmacotherapy in the treatment of vulvodynia pain. J Sex Med 2013;10(10):2497–505.

31. Spoelstra SK, Borg C, Weijmar Schultz WC. Anticonvulsant pharmacotherapy for generalized and localized vulvodynia: a critical review of the literature. J Psychosom Obstet Gynaecol 2013;34(3):133–8.

32. Tommola P, Unkila-Kallio L, Paavonen J. Surgical treatment of vulvar vestibulitis: a review. Acta Obstet Gynecol Scand 2010;89(11):1385–95.

33. Woodruff JD, Genadry R, Poliakoff S. Treatment of dyspareunia and vaginal outlet distortions by perineoplasty. Obstet Gynecol 1981;57(6):750–4.

34. Goetsch MF. Patients' assessments of a superficial modified vestibulectomy for vestibulodynia. J Reprod Med 2008;53(6):407–12.

35. Goetsch MF. Surgery combined with muscle therapy for dyspareunia from vulvar vestibulitis: an observational study. J Reprod Med 2007;52(7):597–603.

Pelvic Floor Physical Therapy for Vulvodynia
A Clinician's Guide

Stephanie A. Prendergast, MPT

KEYWORDS

- Vulvodynia • Vestibulodynia • Dyspareunia • Pelvic floor dysfunction
- Pelvic floor physical therapy

KEY POINTS

- Most women with complaints of vulvar pain have pelvic floor dysfunction.
- Pelvic floor screenings can be easily incorporated into a gynecology examination to identify pelvic floor dysfunction.
- Successful treatment plans for vulvodynia are multimodal and include pelvic floor physical therapy.

INTRODUCTION OF NEW NOMENCLATURE

In 2003, the International Society for the Study of Vulvovaginal Disease (ISSVD) defined vulvodynia as 'vulvar discomfort, most often described as burning pain, occurring in the absence of relevant visible findings or a specific, clinically identifiable, neurologic disorder'. This terminology served to acknowledge vulvar pain as a real disorder but fell short of classifying the syndrome as anything more than idiopathic pain. At that time, little was known about the pathophysiologic mechanisms that cause vulvodynia and treatment options were limited. Over the past decade, researchers have identified several causes of vulvodynia as well as associated factors/impairments. This identification resulted in the need to develop a new classification system to guide physicians toward better diagnosis and treatment. Last year the ISSVD, the International Society for the Study of Women's Sexual Health, and the International Pelvic Pain Society came together to review the evidence and publish the 2015 Consensus Terminology and Classification of Persistent Vulvar Pain and Vulvodynia. Individuals from the American College of Obstetrics and Gynecology, American Society for Colposcopy and Cervical Pathology, and the National Vulvodynia Society also participated.[1]

Pelvic Health and Rehabilitation Center, 11500 West Olympic Boulevard, Suite 440, Los Angeles, CA 90064, USA
E-mail address: stephanie@pelvicpainrehab.com

Obstet Gynecol Clin N Am 44 (2017) 509–522
http://dx.doi.org/10.1016/j.ogc.2017.05.006
0889-8545/17/© 2017 Elsevier Inc. All rights reserved.

obgyn.theclinics.com

The 3 societies reviewed the evidence and determined that persistent vulvar pain caused by a specific disorder can be categorized into 7 different groups, with vulvodynia as a distinct separate entity of vulvar pain not caused by a specific disorder (**Box 1**). In addition, 8 factors/impairments were shown to be associated with vulvodynia, though the research does not yet support if these factors are a cause or an effect (**Box 2**). The final consensus and conclusion was that "vulvodynia is not one disease but a constellation of symptoms of several (sometimes overlapping) disease processes, which will benefit best from a range of treatments based on individual presentations." Although each case of vulvodynia is different, there is one underlying common component in these women that can cause significant pain and functional limitations: the pelvic floor muscles, which are the focus of this article.

PREVALENCE OF MUSCULOSKELETAL IMPAIRMENTS IN WOMEN WITH VULVODYNIA

When clinicians think of pelvic floor disorders, low-tone disorders associated with stress urinary incontinence, pelvic organ prolapse, the peripartum period, and menopause often come to mind. The treatment solution is often saying *do your Kegels*. Over the past 2 decades, numerous, repeated studies have concluded that high-tone or hypertonic pelvic floor muscles are associated with pelvic pain disorders and dyspareunia, including vulvodynia.[2–5] Although it may be less common to think of high-tone or overactive pelvic floor disorders, these disorders affect roughly 16% of women. Currently it is estimated that 10 million women have chronic pelvic pain; less than 70% will receive a proper diagnosis, and 61% will remain undiagnosed.[5] Reissing and colleagues[6] reported that 90% of women diagnosed with provoked vestibulodynia demonstrated pelvic floor dysfunction. In 2015, Witzeman and colleagues[7–9] conducted a proof-of-concept study to determine mucosal versus muscle pain sensitivity in women with provoked vestibulodynia. They concluded mucosal measures alone may not sufficiently capture the spectrum of the clinical pain report

---

Box 1
2015 Consensus terminology and classification of persistent vulvar pain and vulvodynia

A. Vulvar pain caused by a specific disorder[a]
   a. Infectious (eg, recurrent candidiasis, herpes)
   b. Inflammatory (eg, lichen sclerosus, lichen planus, immunobullous disorders)
   c. Neoplastic (eg, Paget disease, squamous cell carcinoma)
   d. Neurologic (eg, postherpetic neuralgia, nerve compression or nerve injury, neuroma)
   e. Trauma (eg, female genital cutting, obstetric)
   f. Iatrogenic (eg, postoperative, chemotherapy, radiation)
   g. Hormonal deficiencies (eg, genitourinary syndrome of menopause [vulvovaginal atrophy], lactational amenorrhea)

B. Vulvodynia: vulvar pain of at least 3 months' duration, without a clear identifiable cause, which may have potential associated factors; The following are the descriptors:
   a. Localized (eg, vestibulodynia, clitorodynia) or generalized or mixed (localized and generalized)
   b. Provoked (eg, insertional, contact) or spontaneous or mixed (provoked and spontaneous)
   c. Onset (primary or secondary)
   d. Temporal pattern (intermittent, persistent, constant, immediate, delayed)

[a]Women may have both a specific disorder (eg, lichen sclerosis) and vulvodynia.
From Bornstein J, Goldstein AT, Stockdale CK. 2015 ISSVD, ISSWSH, and IPPS Consensus terminology and classification of persistent vulvar pain and vulvodynia. J Lower Gen Tract Dis 2016;20(2):128; with permission.

Box 2
2015 Consensus terminology and classification of persistent vulvar pain and vulvodynia, appendix of associated factors

Appendix: potential factors associated with vulvodynia[a]
- Comorbidities and other pain syndromes (eg, painful bladder syndrome, fibromyalgia, irritable bowel syndrome, temporomandibular disorder)
- Genetics
- Hormonal factors (eg, pharmacology induced)
- Inflammation
- Musculoskeletal (pelvic muscle overactivity, myofascial, biomechanical)
- Neurologic mechanisms: central and peripheral (neuro-proliferation)
- Psychosocial factors (eg mood, interpersonal, coping, role, sexual function)
- Structural defects (eg, perineal descent)

[a]The factors are ranked in alphabetical order.
Adapted from Bornstein J, Goldstein AT, Stockdale CK. 2015 ISSVD, ISSWSH, and IPPS consensus terminology and classification of persistent vulvar pain and vulvodynia. J Lower Gen Tract Dis 2016;20(2):128; with permission.

---

in woman with provoked vestibulodynia, which is consistent with the success of physical therapy in this population. Although it is not routine for a gynecology examination to include a screening of the pelvic floor muscles, tissues, and nerves, a simple screening can be a useful tool and is described in this article. Identifying musculoskeletal dysfunction will enable gynecologists to determine if their patients are good candidates for pelvic floor physical therapy. Additionally, this article describes the components of physical therapy evaluation and reviews the evidence for physical therapy treatment.

PELVIC FLOOR ANATOMY AND PHYSIOLOGY

The pelvic floor muscles are grouped as superficial or deep. The superficial muscles, also known as the urogenital diaphragm, include the bulbospongiosus, ischiocavernosus, the superficial transverse perineal muscles, and the urethral and anal sphincter muscles. These muscles, shown in **Fig. 1**, are more commonly associated with vulvar pain syndromes.[6] The deep layer consists of the levator ani muscle group and the coccygeus. Additionally, the obturator internus and piriformis muscles play a role in pelvic floor muscle function. The pelvic floor has unique innervation and is never completely at rest, which helps us maintain continence but also comes with certain consequences in the face of dysfunction and treatment.

The pelvic floor muscles are innervated by sacral nerve roots, the pudendal nerve, and the levator ani nerve. There is slight controversy over specific innervation of the pelvic floor muscles, and naturally anatomic variance exists. For the sake of this article, the author discusses the anatomy in a manner that is clinically relevant. The pudendal nerve arises from S2 to 4 nerve roots and is responsible for sensation for part of the vulva and vestibule, distal portion of the urethra and rectum, anal sphincter, perineum, vaginal mucosa, and pelvic floor muscles. It is a unique, mixed nerve with autonomic fibers in addition to its sensory and motor components. Pudendal neuralgia can be a cause and/or effect of pelvic floor dysfunction and vulvodynia and must be considered for an accurate differential diagnosis. Additionally, branches of the genitofemoral, ilioinguinal, iliohypogastric, and posterior femoral cutaneous nerves are other important nerves for genital pain because of their sensory distribution (**Fig. 2**).

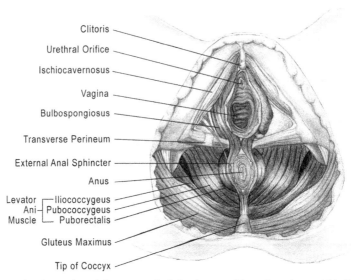

Fig. 1. Superficial muscles of the urogenital diaphragm. (*From* Prendergast SA, Rummer EH. Pelvic pain 101. In: Prendergast SA, Rummer EH, editors. Pelvic pain explained: what everyone needs to know. Lanham (MD): Rowman & Littlefield Publishers; 2016. p. 4; with permission.)

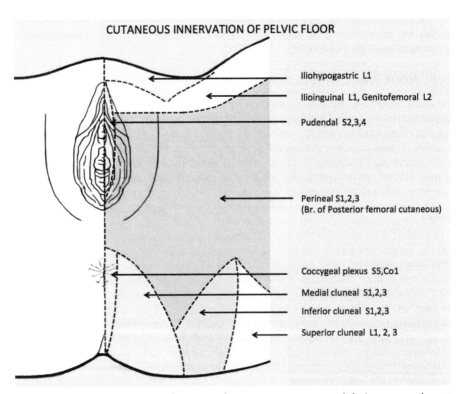

Fig. 2. Peripheral pelvic nerves. (*From* Jacobs D. Dermo neuro modulating: manual treatment for peripheral nerves and especially cutaneous nerves. 2016; with permission.)

The muscles of the pelvic floor and their fascia are responsible for urinary, bowel, and sexual function as well as support of the pelvic viscera. When these muscles become hypertonic, the symptoms that result are as numerous as their normal functions and manifest in a variety of combinations (**Box 3**).

The pelvic floor muscles and nerves can become impaired in several ways; the first step to understanding how patients developed pelvic pain is to begin with their history.

Although we know pelvic floor dysfunction is associated with vulvodynia, the pathophysiological processes are not fully understood. It is suspected that musculoskeletal dysfunction could arise via several different mechanisms (**Box 4**).

PATIENT HISTORY

As previously mentioned, multiple triggers of vulvodynia have been identified. The history is the perfect time to try to identify specific contributing factors to the development of vulvodynia in a symptomatic person. **Box 5** lists the general categories of questions that are often included in a physical therapy evaluation. In addition to mechanistic questions, the physical therapy evaluation also includes a screening for central nervous system hypersensitivity/central sensitization. All pathophysiologic factors, whether a trigger of vulvodynia or a consequence of it, need to be taken into account to formulate an individualized assessment and successful multimodal treatment plan.

PHYSICAL THERAPY EXAMINATION

The information gathered from the history will help guide the physical therapy examination. A primary focus of this article is the pelvic floor muscles, and this component of the physical therapy examination can be replicated by the general gynecologist. In addition to the pelvic floor examination, physical therapy evaluations also include other relevant external static and dynamic components to identify specific impairments. **Box 6** lists common components of the external physical therapy examination while the next section describes the internal examination in more detail.

The external musculoskeletal system can cause as much havoc on the vulva as the pelvic floor muscles, tissue, and nerves. Connective tissue restrictions can lead to local and referred pain, decreased blood flow, underlying muscle dysfunction, and tissue hypersensitivity.[10] Myofascial trigger points can also cause local and referred pain, proprioceptive dysfunction, and central sensitization.[11] The role and existence of myofascial trigger points are currently being debated in the medical community though numerous studies have suggested they play a significant role in pain syndromes. A myofascial trigger point is defined as a hyperirritable group of muscles

---

Box 3
Common symptoms of hypertonic pelvic floor muscles

- Urinary urgency, frequency, hesitancy, pain
- Constipation, difficulty and/or painful bowel movements
- Dyspareunia
- Pain with sitting
- Vulvar, perineal, anal and/or clitoral itching, pain or burning
- Anorgasmia or pain with orgasm
- Clothing and exercise intolerance

Box 4
Possible causes of pelvic floor musculoskeletal dysfunction

1. Higher muscle tension as a reflexive protective response to pain of different origins (neuropathic, infectious, and so forth)

2. Higher muscle tension in general (genetic predisposition)

3. Volitional and/or subconscious pelvic floor guarding in response to stress and/or pain

4. Biomechanical origins (labral tear, sacroiliac joint dysfunction, motor discoordination, overuse, repetitive strain, chronic constipation/straining/labor or compression injuries)

5. Viscerosomatic reflex (gynecologic disease, irritable bowel syndrome, vaginal or urinary tract infections)

6. Inflammation of peripheral nerves

7. Central nervous system hypersensitivity/overactivity

---

fibers that remain in a contracted state at rest. The typically occur at the motor end plate of peripheral nerves. They can be identified by palpation, needle electromyogram (EMG), and possibly by 3-dimensional ultrasound imaging.[11] Neural irritation can stem from mechanical compromise including connective tissue and muscle dysfunction; it can be a cause of tissue and muscle dysfunction and can independently cause pain anywhere in its distribution. Nerves can also be sensitized by repetitive infections or other metabolic processes. Research has also shown a correlation between sacroiliac joint dysfunction, labral tears, and pelvic pain; therefore, these areas also need to be screened.[12,13] The next component of the physical therapy is the skin inspection of the vulva and transvaginal examination, which is described with more detail.

Box 5
Evaluation questions: general categories

1. General lifestyle and timing: When did your symptoms start and what do you think caused it? What makes it better and what makes it worse? Have you had pain from first vaginal insertion or did this develop over time? Where is the location of this pain and other body pains?

2. Urologic: Do you have a history of urinary tract infections? How many time in a day and at night do you void? Is it difficult to start your stream? Do you have pain before, during, or after voiding and if so, where? How long do the symptoms last? Do you ever leak urine?

3. Gynecologic: Do you have a history of vaginal infections? How many culture-proven infections have you had in the past year? Do you have a history of other venereal or gynecologic diseases? Do you have a history of pregnancies, deliveries, or surgeries? What is your menstrual history and frequency? What is your oral contraceptive history?

4. Gastrointestinal: Do you experience abdominal pain, bloating, constipation, hemorrhoids, fissures, or anal pain or itching?

5. Sexual: Do you have pain with intercourse or arousal? Is it superficial or deep? Do you have clitoral pain? Are you able to orgasm? Do you experience genital swelling with stimulation or bleeding or itching?

6. Central sensitization screening

7. What is your past surgical and medical history?

> **Box 6**
> **External physical therapy physical examination for pelvic pain**
>
> - Soft tissue structures:
>   - Connective tissue evaluation of the abdomen, trunk, bony pelvis, legs
>   - Myofascial trigger point/hypertonus evaluation of the pelvic girdle muscles
>   - Neural irritation/dynamics testing of the ilioinguinal nerve, posterior femoral cutaneous, genitofemoral nerve, sciatic nerve
> - Skeletal structures:
>   - Sacroiliac joints
>   - Hip joint
>   - Lumbar spine
> - Biomechanics/motor control evaluation

SKIN INSPECTION AND INTERNAL EXAMINATION
Skin Inspection

- Vulva skin coloring, atrophic or dermatologic changes, fissures
  - This inspection is important to determine if patients need a referral to a vulvo-vaginal dermatologist and further workup or treatment as described in other articles.
- Mobility of clitoral hood, size of clitoris
  - The clitoris should be the size of the head of a Q-tip; the clitoral hood should move easily, without pain, to expose the organ. Reduction in the size of the head of the clitoris can indicate hormonal insufficiencies from oral contraceptive pill use, hormonal suppressive therapies, or menopause. Issues with mobility of the clitoral hood can stem from dermatologic diseases, infection, or connective tissue issues.
- Perineal movement with concentric contraction (squeeze) and Valsalva movement (push)
  - Pelvic floor muscles of normal length should shorten with an attempted contraction and relax or let go at a similar speed. If the muscles do not shorten, it could be because they are already in a shortened position because of a contracture or because patients lack motor control. Impaired muscles show little movement, and they may not relax after contracted or they may relax slowly.
  - If no movement occurs during the Valsalva or push motion, patients may have impaired pelvic floor motor control. It is not common that muscles in a nulliparous woman with pain are at normal or overlengthened positions, though this can occur in women with chronic constipation, vaginal deliveries, and advanced age.
- Vestibule inspection and Q-tip test
  - The inspector notes erythemia and the integrity of the tissues. The Q-tip test is done by lightly touching the vestibule and documenting the location and severity of pain levels. This test is often painful for patients and can sensitize them for the remainder of the examination. If you notice severe redness and they have unprovoked pain, it may make sense to limit the number of areas touched or skip the Q-tip test because it is obvious they have pain.
- Reflex testing: anal wink, clitoral

Internal Pelvic Floor Muscle Examination

- Note: If the vestibule is erythematous and/or very painful on the Q-tip test, it is helpful to be cognizant of this area and avoid unnecessary pressure on this region while accessing the pelvic floor muscles and nerves. If it has already been observed that there is little movement during the requested voluntary movement and the vestibule is erythematous and/or very tender, it is likely that a pelvic floor disorder is contributing to the patients' pain and a physical therapy evaluation is warranted. Therefore, it may be reasonable to stop the examination there. If you think patients can tolerate further examination, the next steps can be performed to gather more information about the musculoskeletal system.

General considerations for the pelvic floor examination

During the digital internal examination, a single gloved, lubricated finger is used. The amount of pressure used is enough to whiten the nail bed when pressing on a table. For the sake of a gynecologic screening of pelvic floor muscles, the examiner is feeling for tone and elasticity while also asking for reports of tenderness and pain. Healthy muscles do not hurt when they are palpated. Repetitive palpation of numerous patients will afford the examiner the knowledge to be able to distinguish tight from normal by touch. Generally speaking, tight muscles are often painful; subjective reports from patients can help guide the interpretation of what the examiner is feeling. We are also examining for motor control. Can patients contract the muscles? Are they already contracted in a state and unable to be volitionally relaxed? Are patients able to Valsalva and move the pelvic floor into a lengthened position if they cannot volitionally relax the muscles? These factors are all factors to keep in mind as the examiner palpates the different pelvic floor muscles listed later. It may be easiest to use the right index finger when examining the muscles and nerves of patients' right pelvis and the left index finger when examining the left.

- Internal pelvic floor palpation
  - Obturator internus and Tinel sign for pudendal nerve irritability: The obturator internus is an external rotator of the hip. This muscle is easily identified by placing a finger in the vagina to a depth just roughly past the second knuckle at 3 or 9 o'clock on the patients' right or left side, respectively, using the ventral aspect of a flat finger. The external hand can be placed on patients' outer knee, asking patients to lightly press into your hand. When patients move in this manner, the obturator internus will contract under your finger, confirming you are on the muscle. This muscle often causes pain at the ischial tuberosities and tailbone as well as contributes to generalized pelvic floor hypertonus. Importantly, the pudendal nerve travels through Alcock canal, which is partially composed of the aponeurosis of the obturator internus. This nerve can be examined for irritability by performing Tinel sign. This test is done by lightly palpating the nerve in the canal. This nerve should feel like a funny bone palpation in normal cases; if light palpation causes sharp, shooting, stabbing pain or burning, the Tinel sign is considered to be positive in this location. If this test is positive, the pudendal nerve can be a factor in patients' vestibulodynia and pelvic pain (**Fig. 3**).
  - Urogenital diaphragm: The urogenital diaphragm contains the bulbospongiosus, ischiocavernosus, and superficial transverse perineum. Reissing and colleagues[6] found this superficial layer displayed in a considerably higher resting tone in patients with provoked vestibulodynia. These muscles can be palpated using a pincer grasp by lightly using the index finger internally and the thumb of the same hand externally up and down the length of the bulbospongiosus, ischiocavernosus, and superficial transverse perineum (see **Fig. 1**). These muscles can be activated by asking patients to do a quick cough or quick flick

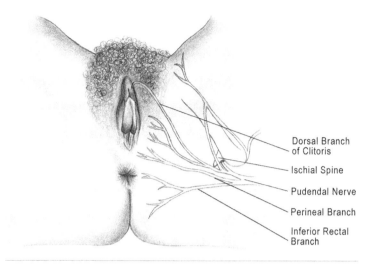

Fig. 3. Pudendal nerve branches. (*From* Prendergast SA, Rummer EH. Demystifying the neuromuscular impairments that cause pelvic pain. In: Prendergast SA, Rummer EH, editors. Pelvic pain explained: what everyone needs to know. Lanham (MD): Rowman & Littlefield Publishers; 2016. p. 43; with permission.)

muscle contraction. They are also involved in orgasm and are often tender and tight in women with painful or absent orgasm. These muscles are considered impaired if they are painful and/or cannot contract or relax.

○ Levator ani muscle group: The pubococcygeus can be found about 1 in into the vagina between 7 and 11 o'clock on the left and 1 and 5 o'clock on the right. The puborectalis can be palpated going slightly deeper and straight down toward the table as it swings around the rectum, at 6 o'clock. The ischiococcygeus can be palpated by going slightly further into the vagina between 4 and 8 o'clock. The overall coordination of this muscle group can be tested by asking patients to squeeze or do a Kegel exercise. The muscles are considered impaired if palpation is painful, if they cannot contract, or if the muscles do not relax after a concentric contraction.

A physical therapy internal examination also includes examination of the vulvar and periurethral connective tissue, palpation of all pudendal nerve branches, the coccygeus, and a more involved investigation of patients' motor control, muscle length, and strength and endurance. Impaired motor control, hypertonus, and tight/short muscles are often the cause of pelvic pain and dysfunction. Physical therapy aims to normalize patients' specific impairments through various treatment techniques described later in this article.

PHYSICAL THERAPY ASSESSMENT AND TREATMENT PLAN

Following the history and the physical examination, a physical therapy assessment and treatment plan is formulated. During this segment of the evaluation, the physical therapist will link the objective findings to specific symptoms and devise a treatment plan to normalize the impairments and to eliminate patients' symptoms. The physical therapist will also discuss short- and long-term goals with patients and create a rough timeline of what to expect. The treatment timeline will vary based on the severity, chronicity, and comorbidities patients present with. In an ideal world, physical therapy appointments occur 1 to 2 times per week for 1 hour for 8 to 12 weeks initially. The constraints of managed care have forced treatment times and duration to often be shorter in many clinical settings than the syndrome requires, so many patients choose to go to an out-of-network provider for longer treatment times and durations.

More often than not, women with vulvodynia have multiple pathophysiologic factors that led to the development of their syndrome. It is critical for their doctors and physical therapist to formulate a differential diagnosis and collaborate on an interdisciplinary treatment plan. This point is best illustrated by case examples and a multimodal treatment algorithm.

CASE EXAMPLES

1. Leah is 30 years old. When she found a new sexual partner last year she developed multiple urinary tract infections that were appropriately treated with antibiotics but unfortunately led to several yeast infections. On evaluation, she presented with high-tone pelvic floor dysfunction; her treatment plan included manual therapy and home exercises to loosen her tight muscles. Leah also consulted with a naturopathic doctor to get to the underlying cause of the repetitive infections. She developed candida in her gut as a result of long-term and repetitive antibiotic use that led to vaginal yeast infections. These infections irritated her tissues and led to persisting muscle hypertonus, which caused further pain. The musculoskeletal dysfunction, inflammation, and the systemic infections were primary causes of Leah's vulvar pain. Her symptoms were successfully treated with manual physical therapy and a pelvic floor down-training home exercise program, a low-sugar and anticandida diet, and a low-dose tricyclic antidepressant.

2. Michelle is 30 years old. Her vulvovaginal pain developed after she was in a car accident. During the car accident, her knees hit the dashboard, causing sacroiliac joint dysfunction. Because of the close relationship between the sacroiliac joint ligaments and the pudendal nerve, she subsequently developed pudendal nerve irritation, which in turn caused a high-tone pelvic floor and constant vulvar burning. Because of the pudendal nerve irritation, Michelle could not initially tolerate physical therapy. She consulted with a pain management physician who prescribed duloxetine (Cymbalta) and performed a pudendal nerve block (peripheral neuropathic treatment), and then she resumed physical therapy. Her physical therapy treatment plan included manual therapy as well as orthopedic treatment strategies of joint mobilization and neuromuscular reeducation for her sacroiliac joint, which was a driving factor in Michelle's case.

3. Gwen is 49 years old and a triathlete. Her vulvar pain started 2 weeks after she started an exercise regime called CrossFit. She noticed the pain when she attempted to have intercourse. On examination, she did not have pelvic floor dysfunction or muscle tenderness, which can be associated with changes in exercise regimes and injuries. Instead, her periods have been irregular and she is in perimenopause. On inspection, her vulvar tissues were thin and atrophic. Her musculoskeletal structures were totally normal. The vulvar pain with intercourse coincided with a change in her exercise routine, but it also coincided with resuming intercourse after a period of inactivity and perimenopause. Her treatment consisted of topical hormonal cream, and she did not need physical therapy.

4. Michelle, who is 24 years old, always had painful periods and was prescribed oral contraceptives at 16 years of age to ease her painful periods. She had a boyfriend from 19 to 21 years of age and was able to enjoy pleasurable intercourse. At 21

years of age, she began using isotretinoin (Accutane) for skin issues. She was still taking oral contraceptives. Subsequently, she began to experience vulvar pain with tampon use; for 2 years she experienced vulvar pain during sex that was becoming increasingly problematic. She then developed a Bartholin cyst that was surgically removed. Following this procedure, she felt daily unprovoked pain at the incision site. On physical examination, she presented with scar tissue at the surgical incision site and also had other identified musculoskeletal findings that likely contributed to her provoked pain. It is plausible that androgen insufficiency from oral contraceptives and Accutane was a contributing cause to the provoked vulvar pain that developed with insertion and that a neuroma secondary to surgery was contributing to the daily unprovoked pain. She was likely a poor surgical candidate because the hormonally sensitive vestibular tissue was compromised from her oral contraceptive pill (OCP) and Accutane use. Her treatment involved cessation of the birth control pill, use of topical and systemic hormonal therapy, surgical excision of the neuroma, and physical therapy. Her case was hormonal, genetic, peripheral neuropathic, and musculoskeletal.

5. Barb is 53 years old and the mother of 2 children, aged 25 and 27 years, delivered vaginally. She underwent a complete hysterectomy and anterior vaginal wall repair for uterine and bladder prolapse. Mesh was used in this repair. Following surgery, Barb developed severe and debilitating vulvar pain. Her pain was caused by peripheral nerve irritation from the mesh, and it was eventually removed. Following the removal of the mesh, she underwent pharmacologic therapy for central nervous system (CNS) hypersensitivity, pudendal nerve blocks, and physical therapy, which resulted in resolution of her symptoms.

ASSESSMENT AND TREATMENT

As shown in the case examples, it is common for patients with similar symptoms to require completely different treatment plans. In order to effectively devise an initial treatment plan, a differential diagnosis and assessment is required. These principles are best highlighted with an interdisciplinary treatment algorithm (**Fig. 4**).

Physical therapists are well positioned to serve as a case manager for patients because of the length of time and repetitive visits over time that they are afforded with patients. It is important that a treatment plan is well coordinated with all of the treating doctors and providers as patients often initially fail or do not tolerate needed treatments. Success lies in the ability to troubleshoot through treatment plan hiccups and find a plan that is tolerated and effective.

In addition to the case management role, the physical therapy treatment plan consists of various combinations of treatment strategies listed in **Box 7**.

EVIDENCE FOR PHYSICAL THERAPY TREATMENT

Physical therapy treatment of vulvodynia is recommended by the American College of Obstetrics and Gynecology.[14] Because of the heterogeneity of the syndrome and the multitude of physical therapy treatment options, the literature often addresses combination approaches to treatment versus individual techniques. This article highlights a few diverse studies.

In 2009, FitzGerald and colleagues[15] published a randomized feasibility trial of 2 methods of manual therapy in patients with chronic pelvic pain. Forty-eight subjects were recruited and randomized to receive either skilled, myofascial physical therapy or global Swedish massage. Each group received 10 weekly 1-hour treatments. Therapist adherence to the treatment protocols was excellent. The global response

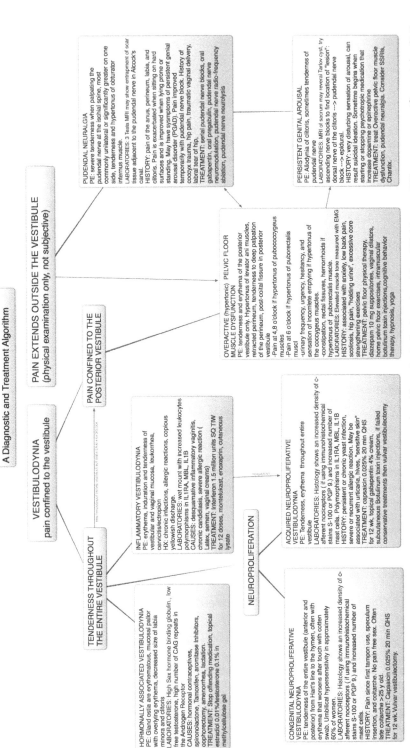

Fig. 4. Vulvar pain and vestibulodynia, a diagnostic and treatment algorithm. CAG, CAG nucleotides; HX, history; PGP, neuron specific protein; QHS, every bedtime; SQ, subcutaneous; SSRIs, selective serotonin reuptake inhibitors. (*Modified from* King M, Rubin R, Goldstein AT. Current uses of surgery in the treatment of genital pain. Curr Sex Health Rep 2014;6(4):253; with permission.)

Box 7
Physical therapy treatment options

1. Manual therapy techniques
   a. Connective tissue manipulation
   b. Myofascial release and myofascial trigger point release
   c. Neural mobilizations
   d. Joint mobilizations

2. Pelvic floor and girdle neuromuscular reeducation

3. Pain physiology education

4. Behavioral and lifestyle modifications to reduce fear/avoidance and catastrophization

5. Peripheral and CNS desensitization strategies

6. Home exercise program development to supplement in-office treatments
   a. Foam rolling
   b. Pelvic floor muscle relaxation exercises (pelvic floor drop)
   c. Stretching when appropriate, strengthening if weak

---

assessment rate was 57% in the myofascial physical therapy group was significantly higher than the rate of 21% in the global therapeutic massage treatment group ($P = .03$).[15]

In another study, Gentilcore-Saulnier and colleagues[16] determined that women with provoked vestibulodynia had higher tonic surface EMG activity in their superficial pelvic floor muscles compared with a control group and a heightened response to painful stimuli when these muscles were subjected to pressure. Physical therapy treatment resulted in less pelvic floor muscle responsiveness to pain, less pelvic floor muscle tone, improved vaginal flexibility, and improved pelvic floor muscle capacity.[16]

In a multimodal study, Goldfinger and colleagues[17] compared the effects of cognitive behavioral therapy (CBT) and physical therapy on pain and psychosocial outcomes in women with provoked vestibulodynia. Twenty women were randomized to receive CBT or physical therapy. Both treatment groups demonstrated significant decreases in vulvar pain during sexual intercourse, with 70% and 80% of the women demonstrating a moderate clinically important decrease in pain (>30%) after treatment.

SUMMARY

Vulvar pain affects up to 20% of women at some point in their lives, and most women with vulvar pain have associated pelvic floor impairments. It is suggested that these impairments are a cause of vulvodynia in some cases, whereas, in other cases, they may be an effect. A quick screening of the pelvic floor muscles can be performed in the gynecology office and should be used when patients report symptoms of pelvic pain. Because of the heterogeneity of the syndrome, successful treatment plans are multimodal and include physical therapy.

HOW TO FIND A PELVIC FLOOR PHYSICAL THERAPIST

Pelvic floor physical therapists can be found through the American Physical Therapy Association' section on women's health (http://www.womenshealthapta.org/pt-locator/) or through the International Pelvic Pain Society's Web site (http://pelvicpain.org/patients/find-a-medical-provider.aspx).

REFERENCES

1. Bornstein J, Goldstein AT, Stockdale CK, et al. 2015 ISSVD, ISSWSH, and IPPS consensus terminology and classification of persistent vulvar pain and vulvodynia. J Sex Med 2016;13(4):607–12.
2. Lev-Sagie A, Witkin SS. Recent advances in understanding provoked vestibulodynia. F1000Res 2016;5:2581.
3. Goldstein AT, Pukall CF, Brown C, et al. Vulvodynia: assessment and treatment. J Sex Med 2016;13(4):572–90.
4. Thibault-Gagnon S, Morin M. Active and passive components of pelvic floor muscle tone in women with provoked vestibulodynia: a perspective based on a review of the literature. J Sex Med 2015;12(11):2178–89.
5. Gyang A, Hartman M, Lamvu G. Musculoskeletal causes of chronic pelvic pain. Obstet Gynecol 2013;121(3):645–50.
6. Reissing E, Brown C, Lord M, et al. Pelvic floor muscle functioning in women with vulvar vestibulitis syndrome. J Psychosomatic Obstetrics Gynecol 2005;26(2): 107–13.
7. Witzeman K, Nguyen RHN, Eanes A, et al. Mucosal versus muscle pain sensitivity in provoked vestibulodynia. J Pain Res 2015;8:549.
8. Jacobs D. Dermo neuro modulating: manual treatment for peripheral nerves and especially cutaneous nerves. 2016.
9. Rummer EH, Prendergast SA. Pelvic pain explained: what everyone needs to know. Lanham (MD): Rowman & Littlefield Publishers; 2016. Available at: https://www.abebooks.com/9781442248311/Pelvic-Pain-Explained-What-Needs-1442248319/plp. Accessed January 25, 2017.
10. FitzGerald MP, Kotarinos R. Rehabilitation of the short pelvic floor. I: background and patient evaluation. Int Urogynecol J Pelvic Floor Dysfunct 2003;14(4):261–8.
11. Travell JG, Simons DG. Myofascial pain and dysfunction: the trigger point manual: lower extremities, vol. 2. Baltimore (MD): Lippincott Williams and Wilkins; 1992.
12. Hartmann D, Strauhal MJ, Nelson CA. Treatment of women in the United States with localized, provoked vulvodynia. J Womens Health Phys Ther 2007;31(3): 34–8.
13. King M, Rubin R, Goldstein AT. Current uses of surgery in the treatment of genital pain. Curr Sex Health Rep 2014;6(4):252–8.
14. Committee opinion no 673 summary. Obstet Gynecol 2016;128(3):676–7.
15. FitzGerald MP, Anderson RU, Potts J, et al. Randomized multicenter feasibility trial of myofascial physical therapy for the treatment of urological chronic pelvic pain syndromes. J Urol 2013;189(1):S75–85.
16. Gentilcore-Saulnier E, McLean L, Goldfinger C, et al. Pelvic floor muscle assessment outcomes in women with and without provoked vestibulodynia and the impact of a physical therapy program. J Sex Med 2010;7(2):1003–22.
17. Goldfinger C, Pukall CF, Thibault-Gagnon S, et al. Effectiveness of cognitive-behavioral therapy and physical therapy for provoked vestibulodynia: a randomized pilot study. J Sex Med 2016;13(1):88–94.

Printed and bound by CPI Group (UK) Ltd, Croydon, CR0 4YY

07/10/2024

01040501-0001